Born in India, the A.H. Khan is a doctor who obtained his basic medical degree in Hyderabad, India, and moved to the United Kingdom (UK) in July 1973. He gained his post-graduate medical qualifications (Anaesthetics and Intensive Care Unit (ICU)) in London and in the Republic of Ireland. He worked in the NHS (National Health Service) when he came to the UK. He has nothing but praise for the NHS.

In addition to his medical qualifications, he has wide general interests. His overall general knowledge, especially in the field of science, is particularly commendable. He has an analytical, logical, unbiased, evidence-based and honest approach to various issues and thus sometimes differs widely from the well-established beliefs.

In addition to this book, the author has written another fact-based fiction novel, *Raisham*, which has already been published.

He has written more fiction and non-fiction. They are awaiting publication.

This book is dedicated to those who 'THINK' and every human being is blessed with this faculty.

Dr. A.H. Khan

STRANGE BUT TRUE

Life experience of a Muslim doctor

AUSTIN MACAULEY PUBLISHERS™

LONDON ∗ CAMBRIDGE ∗ NEW YORK ∗ SHARJAH

A CIP catalogue record for this title is available from the British Library.

ISBN 9781528936187 (Paperback)
ISBN 9781528936194 (Hardback)
ISBN 9781528968591 (ePub e-book)

www.austinmacauley.com

First Published 2022
Austin Macauley Publishers Ltd®
1 Canada Square
Canary Wharf
London
E14 5AA

I am grateful to Barrister Abdus-Saleem Quraishi; my wife, Mrs Mahjabeen Khan; and my children, for discussing various issues and giving me their valuable opinion. I am also grateful to Mr. Akram Sattar for his technical assistance.

Table of Contents

Part One

Preface

I am a medical doctor, and for about 48 years, I have worked in hospitals. Out of these, about 43 years were in the UK, in operation theatres, in intensive care units (ICU), in labour wards and resuscitation rooms of A & E (Accidents & Emergency) departments. I have worked in teaching hospitals as well as in District hospitals. I have nothing but praise for the NHS (National Health Service) and the welfare system in the UK.

As a Muslim, I have studied Islam (and other religions) and have been a regular attendee in various mosques.

I am writing this book because I feel passionate about my thinking, my feelings, and my views. I also feel that I have "something" positive and constructive to give back to the world and to this country, which has given me so much.

For more than sixty years, I have been listening to the imams of the mosques and other religious speakers, known as "scholars", in Friday prayer sermons, during Ramadan and on other occasions. I have also been reading various books written by "scholars" of Islam. They say many good things, but I still find so many flaws in their speeches and writings that I felt strongly that I must write this book.

In this book, I have also written about various incidences which were related to my work in the hospitals. I think that these are of general interest to the public.

The incidences (chapters) are not arranged in an organised way as one would find in a traditional book. Instead, short incidences are put together under one chapter, and long incidences, where more is to be written and discussed, are under different chapters.

There are eight types of topics mingled together.

Six are those that occurred in the operation theatres, ICUs, labour wards, resuscitation rooms in A & E departments and hospital wards and clinics.

The seventh is related to the mosques and Muslim scholars.

The eighth is miscellaneous incidences of general interest.

All the incidences are true. I have changed the names of the people and places because the purpose of the book is not to name and shame the people or defame/degrade anyone or challenge someone's beliefs or way of life, but to highlight some points.

My memories expand from 1954 till 2021, when I wrote this book. With time many things have changed. What was "unacceptable, not the norm, frowned upon" in the 1950s/60s/70s etc., is quite acceptable in society now. If I have written something which someone in today's world, in 2021 finds offensive, biased etc., please remember that I wrote this in view of what was the norm at the time of that incident, how people reacted at that time.

As a Muslim, I have given quotes from the holy Quran and other Islamic literature, but people of other faiths can find similar quotes from their books as the general principles of all the religions are the same.

Dr Azhar H Khan   August 2021
M.B.B.S. (India)
D.A. (London) F.F.A.R.C.S. (London and Republic of Ireland)

Foreword

I know Dr. Azhar for a considerable long time. He is very well educated, comes from a respectable and educated family. His father occupied a higher position in the hierarchy of the educational services of the state of Hyderabad in India.

From the beginning I notice that Dr. Azhar has a thinking mind, does not accept anything at its face value, and knows his limits.

In addition to his specific knowledge in his specific field of medicine, he has very wide general knowledge in the field of sciences and other subjects. His comments on various topic are with an analytical, evidence-based mind. With a logical discussion, he comes out with points which are mostly overlooked by others.

His recently published (May 2021) novel, *Raisham* is a fact- based fiction with many Islamic principles, psychological points, and points of human nature, told in a story form.

Dr. Azhar's present book, Strange but true, Life experience of a Muslim doctor, is a collection of his observations and experiences as a Muslim and as a doctor. As a Muslim, he comments on people's beliefs in religion and their practice, particularly in the Muslim community.

Dr. Azhar's work makes a departure from some stablished beliefs in the Muslim community. This is an exploration towards studying in perspective some of the important issues relating to day-to-day life. This is an incisive, orientated work and does involve some interpretations of the revealed knowledge which attempts to interpret and resolve some of the contradictions.

This work is bound to induce fresh thinking, leading to some balanced assessment on various issues mentioned in the book. The discussions are illuminating and incisive, interpretations are creative and persuasive.

In chapter 15, Ok … OK but no heart, he comments on some Muslims' practice to refuse donating organs for transplant but are ready to take.

In chapter 13, Women suffer in every community, he points out about the women's suffering against the general principles of humanity.

In chapter 10, How, why, when where, what, he mentions that most contemporary religious leaders of Islam are unaware of the importance of science and technology.

Every chapter of this book is worth reading, although dealing with complex and controversial matters, this book is extremely readable and absorbing. Some of his other work is awaiting publication.

I wish him well for his sincere efforts for his creative work.

A S Qureshi

Saleem Qureshi, Barrister-at-law,
Lincoln's Inn, London. September 2021

Chapter One

47 Short Stories (Like the Rest of the Book, all are Strange but True)

Below are some personal incidences, from my childhood, in 1950s India till I retired, in 2016 in the UK. I think they are of general interest to everyone. Most are medically related; some are Islamic-oriented, and others are of general interest.

1. Woman in a pedal rickshaw

In the early 1960s, I was a first-year medical student in Gandhi Medical school, Hyderabad, India.

Much of the time of first- and second-year medical students was spent in the dissection hall, where the students dissected the real dead bodies, as per the syllabus.

The human brain is a very complicated organ and needs a very deep and thorough study. Therefore, it was not included in the first-year syllabus. However, I became interested in finding out if there was an anatomical difference in the male and female brain. The only way to find out was to actually dissect the brains of male and female dead bodies and compare them. As there was no time during the weekdays, I obtained permission from my Anatomy tutor to use the dissection hall on Sundays. I told him what I wanted to do, i.e., dissect the male and female brains to find out any anatomical differences between them. I used to go to the medical college early on Sundays, ask the caretaker to open the dissection hall (In return, I used to give him breakfast money). I used to sit among 25-30 dead bodies, dissecting out their brains.

Needless to say, I could not find any anatomical difference between male and female brains. Now (2021), after years in medicine, I know that we still do not fully understand the functions of the human brain. There was no concept of "neuro-plasty" in the 1960s. The standard teaching was that there was "no regeneration" in the brain tissues. Now we know that the neurons and axons (brain cells and their connections) can survive after the age of 25 and given the right circumstances, they do make new connections. We were taught about the physical diseases of the brain like Epilepsy, Parkinson's disease, Head injury/brain injury, but not how to keep the brain (mind) sharp and avoid diseases like dementia, Alzheimer's etc.

On one Sunday morning, I was in the dissection hall at about 8 am. The caretaker had gone somewhere. I was the one and only person in the entire medical school building, sitting in the dissection hall, surrounded by dead bodies, cutting out their brains. Around 11 a.m., I saw the caretaker coming into the school building, in a pedal rickshaw, with a woman sitting next to him. The woman was wearing a green saree and a yellow blouse. As the rickshaw came near to the dissection hall, I saw that the woman was sleeping and was resting on the shoulder of the caretaker. All kinds of thoughts came to my mind; is the caretaker up to something? Has he drugged the woman? Is he a woman "trafficker?" When the rickshaw stopped at the entrance of the dissection hall, the caretaker called me to help him. Then I realised that he brought a dead woman to be used in the dissection hall. We brought the woman's body into the "embalm" room, took off her clothes, infused the formalin into her body (through the left femoral vein) and…two days later, I was dissecting her body.

Obviously, in those days, either there were no regulations for transporting a dead body, or the caretaker ignored them. In Hyderabad, in those days, there was no scarcity of homeless people who lived on the streets. When they died, nobody claimed their bodies, and they served a very useful purpose of educating the medical students. They lived a poor and lonely life, but in their deaths, they served humanity.

In the 1960s, I was an immature, 1st-year medical student coming from a conservative society, but even today, I feel bad for taking the woman's clothes off. Would she have allowed me (us) to do so in her lifetime? If she had relatives, would they have allowed me (us) to do so? Of course not. Did she pay the price of being poor and homeless? Yes. Did she not deserve a decent burial? Yes, she did. Then I think of hundreds of dead bodies that come into the dissection hall. They all need decent burial, but they do not get it because they are poor.

2. Only my husband can...

In an A & E department in a Kent (England) hospital, I had a woman with quite a bad injury to her leg. She was brought by an ambulance at about 2 p.m. Her leg was swelling fast. She needed surgery quite urgently. I noticed that she had a metal ring in her 2nd left toe. I told her that the ring needed to come out and we were going to cut it. She said that the ring was placed on her toe by her husband when she got married about ten years ago. It was a religious symbol and only her husband could remove it. I told her that it was necessary to remove the ring urgently otherwise it was going to cause irreversible damage to her leg. She was still adamant that only her husband could remove it. I asked her where her husband was. She said he was working. In those days, there were no mobile phones. I got her husband's office number, rang him, and asked him to come to the hospital to remove the ring. He said he could not leave work. I got his permission, on the phone, to remove the ring, had to get another witness, and only then we managed to cut the ring. Her leg was saved.

If I could not have found her husband, she could have been adamant not to remove the ring and could have lost her leg.

3. How much...Will I...?

In the same A & E department, I was doing an afternoon duty. Around 3 p.m., the ambulance brought a car accident victim. The patient was rushed to the resuscitation room. He was very seriously injured. Upon taking the patient's history, he turned out to be an American tourist who was in the UK with his wife. The wife was also in the car, but she was not hurt. She was waiting outside the resuscitation room.

Despite our best efforts, the patient did not survive. As I was the senior-most doctor in the team, it was left to me to break the news of his death to his wife. I took a nurse with me and came out of the resuscitation room. I told the wife that we were very sorry that we could not save her husband. The first thing which she said was, "How much compensation will I get, Doctor?"

4. In the morgue at 2 a.m.

I was working in Greenock, in Scotland, in the early 1980s. One of the patients in the ward was not "going to make it," i.e., was expected to die soon, within hours. I was on call that night and left the ward around 8 p.m. Around 10 p.m. I was sleeping in my room when the sister in charge rang me and said that the patient had died. I asked her if I had to come and write the death certificate. She said that there was no need to go to the ward at that time of the night and write the certificate as the relatives were going to collect the body two days later. I could write the certificate in the morning. She sent the body to the morgue.

Around 2 a.m., she rang again saying that the relatives had changed their mind and were going to collect the body in the morning around 7 a.m. She asked me to come to the ward and write the death certificate. I went to the ward and as I was about to write the death certificate, she told me that I should not write the certificate without examining the body. I told her that she examined the body and that was not enough. She said that legally it should be examined by the doctor who writes the certificate. I asked her, "does this mean I go to the morgue at this time, 2 a.m. and examine the body?" Her answer was "yes."

Morgues and post-mortem rooms are kept cold, and they are usually at the back of the hospitals in lonely, deserted places where not many people go even in the daytime. Going there at 2 a.m., on my own, in December was a spooky experience for me. I could have easily roamed around for half an hour, come back to the ward, and told the sister that I had examined the body. I did not do this, because:

a) I did not want to tell a lie, and;
b) I had recently come back from an examination, where the examiner asked me how to differentiate between a dead person and a person in a deep coma, where even a pulse cannot be felt, and heart sounds are not audible either. There have been cases like this. With this in mind, I had to go to the morgue and examine the body.

So, at 2 am, I went to the morgue, on my own, opened the door and was looking for the register in which it was recorded as to which (dead person) is in which box. I could not find the register and the only way to find out where my "deceased" person was located, was to pull out every single box, open the white sheet tied over the head of the deceased person and see his face. There were about 20 boxes. After opening about 15 boxes, I finally found my patient. I knew him very well, so I recognised him by his face. Now I had to examine him to make sure that he was dead and was not in a deep coma. I pulled out the box completely, undid the white sheet top to bottom, examined the body, did some tests (brain stem death tests) and I was quite sure that he was dead. All this took about an hour, in the furthest part of the hospital, on a cold night, all by myself. At 3 a.m., I left the morgue, went to the ward, and wrote the death certificate. I went back to my room and slept for the rest of the night.

Related strange but true stories:

A). 01-12-2017, B.B.C. red button service: In India, in a private hospital, a new-born baby was declared dead by the doctors. The parents took the body and went to the burial place. As they were about to bury the baby, they felt some movement in the cloth in which the baby's body was wrapped. They opened the cloth. The baby was moving. He was rushed back to the hospital.

Questions were raised about the quality of the private hospitals, which are very expensive.

B). In the 1950s, in Hyderabad, India, I read an article in an Urdu health journal.

In Delhi, it was December and the weather was cold.

An Unani doctor (Hakeem) was sitting in his clinic. In his break from his clinic, he was looking at the road. A funeral procession was passing by, quite close to his clinic. The body was wrapped in white sheets with fresh flowers laid on the body. The Hakeem had his suspicion. He stopped the funeral procession, asked some questions as to when the person died, did he die at home, when the flowers were laid down on the body, and then said that the body was "alive."

The body was taken back to the hospital, where it was found that the person was in a deep coma due to uncontrolled diabetes. Apparently, the patient was declared "dead" at home by the relatives.

The Hakeem was asked how he worked out that the body was alive.

He said that if the body was dead, the flowers should have been fresh because "a dead body is cold."

However, Hakeem noticed that the flowers were fading away; they did not look fresh, although the relatives said that they had put fresh flowers on the body.

Hakeem's conclusion was that the body must have been alive and therefore "warm," and it is the warmth of the body that made the flowers "fade away."

It was a happy ending for the relatives.

In 1950s India, the registration of deaths, births and marriages were not as strict as they are now. With home deliveries, deaths at home and marriages at home, it was impossible to keep a record.

C). In 1970, I had just passed my M.B.B.S. exam. I was doing the house job in medicine in the Gandhi Hospital, Secunderabad, India. One early morning, I was called by the ward nurse to see a patient who was "not waking up." After examining her, I declared her "dead." The consultant (Civil Surgeon) came for the ward round at 8 a.m. I told him about the "dead" patient. He examined the patient, did the blood test for sugar. The sugar was seven times above the maximum normal limit. After infusing the insulin and electrolyte fluids, the patient woke up. She was in a diabetic coma; HHS (Hyperosmolar, Hyperglycaemic State).

5. "Is he dead? Not yet?"

A patient was dying, and he had given his consent to donate his eyes (corneas) for transplant purposes. The recipient was informed that the corneas would be available whenever the patient (the donor) dies, so that he (the recipient) would be ready to come to the hospital. The relatives of the patient (donor) were hoping against hope and praying that he won't die, whereas the recipient and his relatives kept ringing the hospital asking when he was going to get the "new" eyes. Essentially the recipient was asking, "Is he dead? Not yet? When is he going to die?"

Some people who are on the waiting list for an organ transplant have an inner desire that someone, somewhere, would die so that their organs could be used for transplant. There have been cases of "*organ trafficking*" in some countries.

In the British Medical Journal (1 May 2021), there is an article about China's "systemic murder of prisoners of conscience for their organs." Also, there is suspicion of organs being taken from the judicially executed prisoners. Also, concern has been raised in the same article about illegal transplantation (transplant tourism) in other countries, including Egypt, India and the Philippines.

Are we selfish? …in desperate conditions, probably we are.

I have read real-life stories where ships were lost somewhere in the sea, people on board ran out of food and started eating their dead fellowmen, or even killed the weaker ones to survive. Also, in the First World War, soldiers drank their own urine to survive.

The psychology of desperation and selfishness is a special subject. I am not a psychologist; I can only quote verses from the Quran. The summary of these verses is that on the day of resurrection, i.e., judgement, man will be ready to give away his parents, his wife, his children and all the wealth he had in the world in return to avoid any punishment. Another verse says, *"On the day of judgement, the "Man" will run away from his brother, from his mother and father, from his wife and from his children. Everyone would be lost in him/her "self."* Surah 80 Verses 34-37.

6. Punctuation marks

Depending on where you put the punctuation mark, the meaning of a sentence can change slightly or dramatically. For example:

a)   Follow the Prophet, not he will lead you astray.
b)   Follow the Prophet not, he will lead you astray.

a and b have quite different meanings. Another example:

c)   Let us eat, Jeremy. (Here, the person is asking Jeremy to eat with him).
d)   Let us eat Jeremy. (Here, the person is telling someone else that they will eat Jeremy).

An English language professor, in his class, wrote the following words on the blackboard:
"A woman without her man is nothing." Then he asked the class to put the punctuation marks in the sentence.

Boys wrote: A woman, without her man, is nothing.

Girls wrote: A woman: without her, man is nothing.

In the mid-1980s, I was working in the Dumfries and Galloway General Infirmary (UK) as a junior doctor (anaesthetic registrar). I had a young man, in his 20s, involved in a car accident. He was very seriously injured. His story was as follows:

Two young men, in their 20s, stole a car and were racing on the A74. The police were chasing them. The driver lost control and crashed into the central barrier on the A74. The driver died on the spot and the other young man was brought to the hospital. We (I and my consultant) took him to the operation theatres, his bones were fixed, other injuries were treated and he was sent back to the ward.

Ten days later, he was brought back to the theatres to remove the steel frame from his leg. The drugs to anaesthetise him were the same as those I had used ten days ago (this was after consulting my consultant anaesthetist). The orthopaedic surgeon started undoing the steel frame from his leg. The patient developed a severe anaphylactic reaction. I called for help. My consultant came in and took over from me. Despite all our efforts, the patient died.

An investigation was launched.

****

Wherever you work (or even in a social circle), you will have some sincere friends, some diplomatic friends (hypocrites) and some clear enemies. This was the case with me in the department/hospital as well. Those who did not like me tried to prove that I made mistakes in using some drugs. However, my consultant went through my notes and was convinced that I was not at fault. The argument between him and the other party was focused on "A" sentence in a medical book, where the punctuation mark made a difference in the meaning. Other medical books were referred to. In one book, the comma was in one place and implemented that a particular drug should not be given. In another book, the comma was in another place, and it was OK to use the drug. How to take the meaning of such different punctuation marks also depends on the reader's intention and what is already in his mind. My consultant successfully argued in my favour saying that my intention was good, and I acted in good faith. The drugs I administered were after discussing with my consultant and I followed his advice.

A few days later, the post-mortem was done, and it emerged that the patient died because of a massive clot in his lung (pulmonary embolism). This clot was sitting in his broken leg and as the steel frame was being removed, it got dislodged and travelled in the bloodstream and got stuck in the main blood vessel in the lung. His death was nothing to do with the drugs I had used—what a great relief.

7. Disciplinary committee

As I have written above, where there are friends, there are enemies.

This happened in a London hospital where I worked for 27 years as a consultant anaesthetist.

Being pregnant and giving birth is a painful process (Surah 46, verse 15, and Surah 31, verse 14). The process of giving birth starts when the woman starts getting labour pains. These pains get more and more severe as the labour progresses. There are ways to relieve these pains. The most efficient one is an injection in the back (epidural).

To do an epidural injection successfully, the mother must be able to sit comfortably, i.e., not shaking, not moving and ideally be pain-free.

I had told the midwives many times to call me to do epidurals "before" the women start getting labour pain. Midwives have an idea when a woman is likely to start having labour pains. The midwives did not stick, all the time, to what I had told them.

I was called to do the epidural on a patient, a non-English lady, who was very distressed with the labour pains. She was unable to sit quietly and comfortably in her bed, even for few seconds. I was unhappy with the situation but still decided to go ahead. When doing the epidural injection, the doctor is working, i.e., giving an injection in the back, very close to the spinal cord and the major nerves supplying the thighs and legs. A slight mistake can damage the spinal cord and the nerves with serious consequences. What is desirable is a quiet, comfortable, and cooperative patient who speaks English. My patient was neither quite nor comfortable nor co-operative nor English speaking. However, I had faced these situations before and was used to handling them. I had given epidural injections in the most uncomfortable and distressed patients who did not speak English.

What was different this time was that the patient's mother and mother-in-law were leaning over my shoulders, one on each side, and shouting to the patient in their language, in a high pitched, harsh voice, trying to calm her down. It felt as if my eardrums were about to burst.

Now the situation was that the patient was sitting on the bed, very distressed and in pain, unable to sit quietly, I was working on her back and the two women were shouting in my ears. Their shouting was becoming unbearable for me to work comfortably and safely. I told the midwife to tell the two women to leave the room. She did so, the two women left, and I completed the epidural injection. Ten minutes later, the patient was pain-free, happily sitting in her bed. A few hours later, she gave birth to a baby boy. All was well.

A few days later, I got a letter from the managers that the midwife had complained against me, saying that I was rude to the patient's relatives. I was called in front of a "disciplinary" committee to explain my behaviour.

As I said earlier, where there are friends, there are foes. Some members in the disciplinary committee were the foes. The reason was I had joined the department recently. They saw me as a threat to their position, their authority and, more importantly, a threat to their private practice. Their leader was a fellow Indian. They tried their best to find me of wrongdoing and get rid of me.

It says in the Quran that no matter what anyone plans, ultimately, what happens is what Allah wills. Surah: 81, last verse.

There were two members of the committee on my side. They both were consultants. One was an English lady, a gynaecologist. She was a very decent, dignified, well respected, straight-forward and quite powerful lady, a true Christian. The other was a Welsh person, in charge of the ICU, very straightforward and fair.

In the Quran, Surah: 57, verse: 27 it says that Allah has ordained kindness and compassion in the hearts of those who follow Jesus.

These two fought in my favour, against my fellow Indians and ultimately, I was cleared of any wrongdoing.

8. Baby in the box

One afternoon, in a London hospital, I was the consultant on call, and I was called to the paediatric resuscitation room.

An eighteen-month-old baby was brought into the room with the history of "baby stopped breathing". There was already an A & E Consultant and other doctors in the room who were doing what was necessary. At my first glance, I realised that the baby was dead. However, since I was not there from the beginning and my first impression could have been wrong, I kept quiet and took the "head-end" to continue the resuscitation process. There was a junior doctor with me. I asked him to put a breathing tube in the baby's windpipe. He did so under my supervision. I checked and the tube was in the right place. The resuscitation process continued but without any positive results. After about 45 minutes, it was decided to abandon the resuscitation and the baby was declared dead. I wrote my notes and went back to the theatres to continue with the day's work.

A few weeks later, I got a letter from the A & E consultant who said that the baby's post-mortem was done, and he died because the breathing tube was not in the right place. This stopped his oxygen supply to his body and that was the cause of his death. Now I was responsible for his death.

I was one million per cent sure that the breathing tube was in the right place and that the baby was dead when he was brought to the hospital. I decided to go into more details of the post-mortem report.

It emerged that the baby's body was transferred in a box from this East London hospital to the Great Ormond Street Hospital (G.O.S.) for the purpose of the post-mortem, as the pathologist in our hospital was not trained to do babies' post-mortem. The breathing tube was not removed from the baby's body. This made my job easy as I knew why the breathing tube was found in the wrong place (food pipe) during the post-mortem.

I successfully argued and demonstrated that when the baby's body was transferred in a vehicle to the G.O.S., there must have been jerks and jolts in the vehicle while it was travelling on the roads. With these movements, the baby's head was moving up and down. As the breathing tube was fixed at the lips, when the head moved backwards, the tube came out of the windpipe and when the head moved forward, the tube took the path of least resistance (principle of physics) and went into the food pipe. With any subsequent movements of the head, the tube kept coming out and going into the food pipe. Going through the notes in detail, I also convinced the A & E consultant that the baby was already dead when brought to the resuscitation room.

My argument was convincing, and I was cleared of any wrongdoing— attention to details paid off.

9. Dr P. Nayak (not the real name)

In the early 1970s, I was working in a London hospital as a junior doctor and was preparing for my first ever exam in the UK. The exam systems in the 1970s in India and in the UK were quite different. I was struggling with my studies, mainly because of the different systems of the exam but also because I was very homesick. I had recently arrived in the UK. With the new country, new weather, no Indian food, a new way of life and work and loneliness, I was having difficulty in adjusting to all these (typical adjustment reaction).

Allah has power over everything. He can make anyone's heart soft for you.

One of my consultants was Dr P. Nayak. One day he saw me in the operation theatres and came to me. He asked me if everything was OK and why I was looking worried. I told him that I was worried about my studies and exam. I told him that I was new in the UK and I had never taken a UK exam before. He went away without saying anything. The next day he came with some books and some old question papers. He told me to study from those books and start writing answers to the questions from the old question papers. He was taking a special interest in my studies. He was putting his own time to teach me, correct my answer papers and giving clues as to the way the British system of examination worked. He was giving me mock viva exams and teaching me various "tricks of the trade." With all his and my efforts, I passed the exam on the first go. Dr Nayak was very happy, did not ask me anything in return, and when I finished my job in that hospital and was leaving, he gave me a big hug and wished me good luck for the future.

Why did Dr Nayak take so much interest in me? Surely, Allah had put that thought in his mind.

It reminded me of the story of Prophet Yousuf (Joseph) in the Quran. When his brothers took him to the jungle and planned to kill him, one of the brothers said not to kill him but to leave him in a well, and hopefully, some passing by caravan would take him. Surely, this thought of leaving Joseph in a well rather than killing him was put in the brother's mind by Allah. This part of the story ends with a verse that says, "*Allah has full power and control over all his affairs, but most people know not*" Surah 12, Verse 21.

Dr Nayak was a Hindu, and yet he helped me...a Muslim. This took my mind to the early 1950s when we were in Gulberga, a town in mid-India. Once, Hindu-Muslim riots erupted in Gulberga. Many people from both sides were killed. Behind our house, a mass grave was dug, and many dead Muslims were "thrown" in that mass grave. When my younger sister saw that, she went into such a shock that she could not speak for three days.

However, during the same riots, there were stories where Muslims saved some Hindus and Hindus saved some Muslims. My father was one of them who sheltered a Hindu boy from his school until the riots died down.

Remembering this and the various verses from Quran where Allah asks you to "*say what is right, do what is right...you will be asked about your deeds*", I have always treated my non-Muslim colleagues and juniors fairly and justly. I preferred Ramgopal over Malik Husain as that was the right thing to do (see chapter 11). I gave good references to some Hindu juniors, as they deserved this. They went on to become consultants.

People's beliefs are their personal matter. Our job is to treat everyone fairly and justly. Remember accountability all the time, every time.

Rioters do not have any religion. The above example where Muslims and Hindus protected each other shows that there are good people in every community. There have been many incidences in the Indian subcontinent where Shias and Sunnis were at each other's throats. I am sure there must be some good people among them who do not support such actions. However, I personally know three "religious" Sunni Muslims, two doctors and one non-medical professional, who have typical Muslim appearance, hold sessions of Quranic teaching and explanations, are highly respected in the society, but privately, they hate Shias and Hindus, and anyone who does not follow their "version" of Islam. The salvation of the entire humanity is in their "version" of Islam.

I want to ask such people one question: "If they need a blood transfusion and the blood is from a Shia or Hindu or anyone else whom they hate, would they refuse to take the blood?" The same question stands for organ transplants.

The Quran gives some basic principles of preaching. "Call people to the path of your Lord with wisdom and with nice, soft, and polite dialogues." Surah: 16, Verse: 125. "If they do not listen, leave them alone. On the day of judgment, Allah will make a final decision as to who was right and who was wrong." Surah: 22, Verse: 17.

10. Should not have done...should have done

In an East London hospital, where I worked for 27 years as a consultant, I defended myself successfully in a coroner's court against the death of a patient who died six hours after having Thyroid surgery.

In another case, in the same hospital, again, I defended myself successfully against the death of a patient who died because of delayed cervical cancer treatment. The consultant gynaecologist was a lady, J.S.M. I am not a gynaecologist or an oncologist (one who treats cancer patients). However, I was dragged into this case, but since it was not my fault, I managed to come out clean.

In my 45 years of experience working in the hospitals, I learnt that in any case of litigation, there are two questions you must come out clean. They are:

a) Have you done something which you should not have done?

b) Have you not done something which you should have done?

Now I am retired, I have more time to think about other things, other than medicine.

Thinking about the two questions above, they are applicable, in general, in this world and in the hereafter.

Quite a few problems we have in this world, as an individual, as a family or as a nation, or even internationally, are because we have done something which we should not have done, or we have not done something which we should have done.

In the hereafter, again, all the questions you will be asked during your accountability will be based on these questions.

Guidance on what one should and should not do in this world is clearly given in the heavenly books. All of them are true and give the same message, especially the last edition, i.e., The Holy Quran.

11. "Do not ask such questions."

It was a Friday prayer time. I went to the mosque in East London. During his sermon, the imam said one Hadis (Prophetic saying), the essence of which was that if a Muslim comes out of his house with the intention of killing another Muslim and the other Muslim also comes out of his house with the intention of killing the first Muslim then they both will go to hell, regardless of who kills and who is killed.

After the prayers, I asked the imam that in view of this Hadis, what was the position of the Muslims who were in two groups in the battle of "Jamal (camel)." (Saudi Arabia year 656). Each group came out of their houses with the intention of killing the other group. Would they all go to hell?

The imam kept quiet for few seconds and then said, "Do not ask such questions."

I would have been a lot happier if he had told me that yes, there must be an answer to your question. Yes, I do not know the answer, but I will investigate. Yes, I will try and find an answer. The Hadis is not wrong, so there must be an explanation.

This is the problem I have seen with most Imams. They give speeches but avoid questions. I have a long list of questions to which I cannot find satisfactory answers.

During my higher medical studies (FRCA) in London, I have attended many courses.

At the end of each day of the course, an "evaluation" form (feedback) is given to all the students (doctors), in which the students have to mark the performance of each lecturer under various headings, like the content of the lecture, its relevance to the course, points the students learnt and most importantly "how can the speaker improve his performance."

Later, in my career, as a consultant, I have given many presentations and adopted this approach. I encouraged the audience, all highly qualified doctors, to "criticise" me in a positive sense so that I could improve myself and give a better talk next time. I expected this approach with our imams but without success. Their approach is: "Don't ask questions, simply believe whatever we say." If you ask questions, it is regarded as disrespect to the speakers and to the writers of the books, from which the speakers take their points.

No man has absolute and perfect knowledge. There is one and only entity who has "all and perfect knowledge," as it says in Surah Yousef (Joseph), Surah: 12, verse: 76. *"Above all those endowed with knowledge, there is one all-knowing, i.e., Allah…*

February 2018. There was an open day in a mosque. I was invited to be a volunteer to guide the visitors, take them to various exhibits and answer their questions. This mosque does not allow women worshipers.

Before the open day, I asked one imam of the mosque, "if the visitors ask me, why are women not allowed to offer their prayers in this mosque? What do I say?"

He did not have an answer to my question.

I asked the same question to another imam of the mosque. He did not have an answer either. He kept looking at me. His face was saying: "Don't ask such questions."

12. Twenty years later

Summary of the two verses of the Quran verses No: 120 and 151 from the 6th Surah.

"Leave all kinds of sins, open and secret. Do not come anywhere near the shameful sins, openly and secretly." This implies mainly to the sins of sexual nature. In today's terms, they are called orders of public indecency. Allah is saying not to commit such sins, openly or secretly.

In the 1960s, in Hyderabad, in India, when I read these verses, a question came to my mind, "Who would do such an act openly? An act of sexual nature?", why Allah is saying to not do such sins of sexual nature "openly" when nobody does this openly?

I kept thinking about it, without an answer. The religious books do not explain this either. Then I got busy with my medical studies and forgot about it.

Twenty years later, I was working in "a" hospital. I lived in the hospital accommodation, which was a big house with seven rooms on the first floor and a big hall on the ground floor. On Friday nights, "parties" were held in the hall with music and dancing and an open bar, etc. Lots of men and women from within the hospital and outside attended these parties. The doctors who were on call for the night, if they were called out at night, they had to pass through the hall where these parties were held.

One Friday night, I was on call and was sleeping in my room. I was called out at around 3 a.m. I had no choice but to pass through the hall where the party was going on. There were quite a few pairs in the hall doing what is called "public indecency." That is where I understood why Allah said, "do not do such acts secretly and *openly*."

13. Ask your father...

I was working in a hospital in Scotland. I was living in the hospital accommodation. My next-door neighbour was Dr Ram Gopal.

One day I told Ram Gopal that I was going to buy a new car and by the 1st of May, it should be with me. 1st of May came and gone, and there was no new car. Ram Gopal asked me what happened. I told him that I was a bit short of money, I would save for two months, then I would buy the new car. Ram Gopal looked at me in a strange way and said, "What is the big deal? Just ask your father-in-law to pay for the car." To me, it was very strange. I have seen this mentality in quite a few Asian Muslims as well. From time to time, we still get news in the Asian newspapers that a woman has been burnt to death or committed suicide because she did not get enough dowry.

Why do we treat women so badly? Even today, in the 21st century, in Asian countries, a girl is a burden on parents. In Hyderabad, India, in the 1960s, a Muslim man who had five daughters said: "I want to line them up and finish them off with a rifle." Yet these girls grew up, got educated, got married and served their father (and mother) till they (parents) died. Even today, those girls pray for the forgiveness of their parents.

"Gender selection" is a fact in Asian countries, although illegal by law. Parents go for abortion when they find that the foetus is a girl.

"For what crime she was killed?" Quran Surah 81, verse 9.

14. Glorifying God...with no common sense

This true incidence is written in volume one of the books, "Sense of life" by Yusuf Islahi Sahib. The book is written in Urdu, so I have translated its' name as "Sense of life."

Yusuf Islahi is a true scholar. He does not say/write any non-sense. His books are worth reading. He writes an incidence in his book as follows:

Somewhere in India, there was a maulvi sahib (Muslim religious man). He was always busy with his religious activities and remembrance of Allah.

One day he and his friend set out from their village to go to some other place. To do so, they had to cross a river. Some parts of the river were "dangerous spots," and those who knew those spots would never cross the river from those spots. Maulwi sahib knew those spots very well, whereas his friend was new to the place and did not know those spots. As they set out from their village, the maulvi sahib started remembering Allah. His intention was to do so uninterruptedly. When they reached the river, the friend jumped into the river to cross it, got into trouble and almost drowned. Some other people ran to his help and saved his life. Maulwi sahib later told the people that he could see that the friend was crossing the river from the dangerous spot. When he was asked why did he not stop the friend? The maulvi sahib's answer was: "I was remembering Allah; I did not want to interrupt it."

This is a true story; I believe it to be true. There are people like this, who would not use common sense, and, in doing so, think that they are doing a great service to Allah.

In my hospital, one doctor would not answer his bleep on a Friday between 1 pm and 2 pm, no matter how urgently he was needed. He did not want to interrupt his Friday prayer. He stopped doing so after a verbal warning. Another doctor was found dozing off at work because he was up most of the night, "praying."

Going by the life of the Prophet (PBUH), he used to shorten his congregational prayers when he heard of children (accompanied by their mothers) crying in the back rows. This is common sense.

This reminds me of another problem my local mosque has. Here ladies are not allowed in the mosques. The management, advised by the imams, won't learn from the life of the Prophet but bring some historical story to prove that women are not allowed in the mosques. How much of this historical event is true? How much of it is adulteration and exaggeration? Only God knows. Even if the entire event was true, it was for that time only, for whatever reason. It should not become a rule forever.

People who are overwhelmed with their religion lose common sense. This is true with all humans regardless of their religion. See the following examples:

a) Few years back, the local MP, an English man, was called to the local mosque in East London to chat with the Muslim community of his constituency. I was particularly invited by the chairman of the mosque committee to attend the meeting (probably to show to the MP that there are educated people in the Muslim community). During the questions and answers sessions, one young man stood up and asked the MP, "In Islam, interest is haram (forbidden). Student loans are based on interest, what are you going to do about it?" I was embarrassed by the question.

Poor MP, surrounded by all Muslims, could not give a credible answer (If I would have been in his place, I would have said, "it is your problem, not the government's."

2020. An imam of the same mosque, who always says in public, that taking out a student loan is haram; as it is based on interest, privately confessed that he has taken student loans for his children's education. So why have this double standard?

b) In September 2018, again, a young worshiper from the same mosque started a petition that student loans are haram in Islam and the government should do something about it. He asked me to sign, but I refused. I told him that if you have a problem due to your faith, it is your personal problem; do not expect the government to solve your problem. If the government decides to give all Muslim students an interest-free loan, everyone else will demand it, quite rightly, otherwise, it becomes very unfair for them.

c) Daily Mail 26/09/2018, page 28: A devout Christian couple has been taken to court in Exeter by the council for not observing the council's planning permission. Their answer was "We are answerable to God only," and they quoted from Bible, Mathew 22:21.

d) I had a lady patient (neither Muslim nor Christian) with neck and limb injuries who insisted that only her husband could remove her religious necklace and the ring on her toe. The husband was not there, and the injured parts were swelling.

e) One of my juniors, an Asian Muslim doctor, was happy to delay the afternoon operation list on a Friday in a London hospital. The list was supposed to start at 1:30 pm; his Friday prayer was going to finish at 2 pm. He was the only Muslim doctor on the team, and he expected everyone to wait till he finished his prayer. As I was the consultant on call, the team approached me. I told him that prayer was his personal problem; he should not delay the operating list.

The approach of an Arab Muslim doctor in the same hospital was quite different. On a Friday, he would complete the morning list and or start the afternoon list on time, even if he missed the Friday prayer. His belief was, "Prayers are my personal problem, I am paid to do a job in time, I can always do my prayers at the end of the list, and at least my earnings will be halal as I am doing my job for the hours I am paid for." I fully agree with him.

Observing, listing to, and reading the Islamic material, I have concluded that Arabs have a much better understanding of Islam than Asians.

f) I have mentioned elsewhere in this book about an African lady who stopped her cervical cancer treatment because her priest, sitting in Africa, was going to pray for her.

g) I know an imam in East London who stopped all his medications for diabetes and high blood pressure because a senior and more knowledgeable Alim (scholar of Islamic studies) told him that he did not have these diseases but was under the bad spell of Jinns. He was told to chant certain words so many hundred times a day. I told him not to stop his medications. A few months later, he died of an intra-cerebral haemorrhage (bleeding inside the brain). He was a qualified and certified scholar of Islamic studies from a well-known Madrasah in India.

Common sense is an essential ingredient to follow the rules and regulations. If you understand the underlying principle behind a rule, you can modify the rule depending on the circumstances. Obedience to parents is a standard teaching in every religion. On three occasions in my life, I refused to obey my father. Later, he realised that he was wrong (parents are humans, they can make a mistake).

15. Take your brain out and put it aside

In a mosque, in London, on two occasions, two non-Muslims came to revert to Islam. After the Shahada (recitation of basic Islamic belief), the imam gave a short speech on the basic principles of Islam. One of the things he said was, "Islam had nothing to do with your brain, i.e., intelligence and thinking. Pointing towards his head," he said, "If you want to follow Islam, take your brain out of your head and keep it aside."

At the end of his speech, I took the imam in a corner, and I asked him why he said that Islam had nothing to do with "brain", i.e., intelligence and thinking. There are so many verses in the Quran in which Allah invites mankind to think, ponder, and use his brain. Maulvi sahib's reply was, "if you start using your brain, you will lose your faith in the unseen."

More explanation of this is given in chapter ten.

No wonder why some Muslims have left Islam, and some reverted Muslims have gone back to their previous religion or lost any faith in God (YouTube and MEND information).

We need a revolution, an overhaul, in our understanding of Islam. This will come only when we take charge of our own "understanding" of Islam by studying (not reading) the Quran and grasp the fundamental concepts.

16. Only after they knew

A). I had a patient, an English man, who was admitted to the hospital with liver problems. During his stay in the hospital, I visited him quite a few times. He was quite free with me and started talking about his personal life. The summary of his life was that he was a "naughty boy" all his life.

He had various investigations done and then we realised that he had a liver tumour, a cancerous one, and it had spread to other organs. He was referred to the cancer specialist. I kept in touch with him and his prognosis. Unfortunately, he was given less than six months to live. He told me that since he had less than six months to live, he wanted to die at home and more so, he wanted to undo all the "bad" things he had done.

He wanted to go back to God with a sin-free soul.

B) In India, one of my relatives was a worldly man. He was very well off, very proud of his wealth and position. He was a doctor. He did not care much about religion. Later in his life, he was diagnosed with pancreatic cancer and was given few months to live. Then he changed. The man, who did not know where the local mosque was, started going there regularly. With time he was getting weaker and weaker. He needed help to take him to the mosque. One day, I was taking him to the mosque, the weather was nice and sunny, but the man was looking very depressed. To cheer him up, I said to him, "Look, it is such a nice sunshine." He looked at me with a sad face, paused for few seconds and said in an incredibly sad tone, "This sun is shining for you. For me, the sun has set, and it is darkness everywhere."

One day, I took him to the mosque. After the congregational prayers, I found him sitting in a corner. I went and sat behind him. He was crying like a child and asking Allah for forgiveness. His cry and prayer for forgiveness were very touching. He died soon after this. I hope Allah has forgiven him.

C) Our neighbour in England was a Nigerian lady. She was not nice to my family and I at all. She herself had many family problems. Her husband had left her. One of her sons was involved in drug dealings. She was taking her frustration out on us because, by the grace of Allah, I had a very stable family. She caused us all sorts of problems.

When we were having some building work done in our house, she created a lot of fuss and obstructions. Any visitors of mine, if he parked his car in front of her house, she would make a lot of fuss.

All this changed when she was diagnosed with breast cancer which had spread all over the body. She was given few months to live. Till she died, she was very nice to us.

D). I had a colleague in London, a lady doctor from Sri Lanka. She was a consultant as well. She hated me. It was a one-sided professional rivalry. She did not miss any chance to create problems for me.

She completely changed when she was diagnosed with terminal cancer, with few months to live.

All the above patients died within their given time.

Comments: We all know that we are going to die at some point in time. Do we have to know when we are going to die to change our attitudes toward others?

17. Muslim lady paediatrician (children's doctor)

Once I met a lady paediatrician in London. When I asked her where did she work? Her answer was: "Nowhere...I do not do any regular job. If I do any regular job, I cannot do my daily prayers on time. Only when I run out of money, then I go and do locum work. With whatever money I get from that locum, I sit at home doing my prayers. When the money runs out, I go and do locum again."

Obviously, this doctor did not understand Islam and its flexibilities. There are thousands of Muslim doctors who do regular jobs, do this honestly, sincerely, and keep themselves up to date with the current medical knowledge in their fields. They are also not behind in religion in any way. If you grasp the fundamentals of Islam, you will work out the flexibilities.

Once, I had two patients for surgery, both with very serious cardiac histories. I did a lot of background preparations, did a lot of research work, got in touch with those who were more experienced than me in dealing with these sorts of cases, and by the grace of Allah, both surgeries were very successful. While doing the background preparations, research work, etc., which took a few weeks and a lot of hard work, I did all my religious duties without any problem, and they did not come in my way to do my work.

If you understand Islam, understand the flexibilities in Islam, then your work will not come in the way of your religious duties and your religion will not come in the way of your work.

I did quite a few complicated cases in my hospital and took full part in the educational activities. The hospital recognised this work by giving me points, with an increase in my pay. All the people who were in the committee to decide who gets the points were non-Muslims. This shows their fairness.

Once I left for the hospital at 7 am. I did my normal work all day. That night, I was the consultant on call. There were many complicated and difficult emergency operations that night. I had to stay in the hospital and help the juniors. By the time I came home, it was 4 am. I had worked for 21 hours continuously. Fajar (dawn) prayer was starting at 5 am. I was in two minds, whether to stay awake for another hour, do my fajar prayer and then go to sleep or sleep now and do fajar prayer whenever I get up.

I remembered three verses from the Quran. In these verses, Allah says, "He has not made the religion, harsh to follow," Surah: 22, Verse: 78. "He wants ease rather than hardship," Surah: 2, Verse: 185. "Do not approach prayer in a state where you do not know what you are saying," Surah: 4, Verse: 43. I had worked for 21 hours continuously in the operation theatres, which is an incredibly stressful job. I was very sleepy. I could have made mistakes in reciting Quran in the Fajar prayer. With all these verses in my mind, I went to sleep and did the fajar prayer when I got up.

If you know the Quran well and use common sense, you will work out the flexibilities.

The doctor who did not answer his bleep every Friday between 1 pm and 2 pm and another doctor who was found dozing off at work (because he was engaged in night prayers) obviously did not understand Islam and did not use common sense.

18. One and only child

One afternoon, I was the consultant on call in a London hospital. I was called to the trauma resuscitation room in the A & E.

A young Hindu boy, about 18 years old, was brought in very bad condition. He was involved in a car accident. He had many broken bones, and it was quite clear that he was bleeding internally as well. If not taken to the operation theatres as soon as possible, he was going to die. The boy's mother was standing at the foot end of the bed, extremely worried as her son was dying in front of her eyes. She kept begging me to do everything possible to save his life. She said, "Doctor Sahib, this is the one and only child I have." She was touching my feet and begging me to do everything to save her son's life. This patient needed urgent X-rays, blood tests and blood X-matching.

The normal procedure is to call a porter to take the patient to the X-ray department. Call another porter to take the blood samples to the blood lab. We rang the porters, and they were busy elsewhere. Normally, people will wait for the porters. I do not know what came to my mind; I, with the help of a nurse, took the patient to the X-ray department. While they were doing X-rays, I ran up and down to organise the blood testing and blood X-matching. As soon as the X-rays were done, rushed the patient to the theatres and started the most urgently needed operation. The boy's life was saved. The boy stayed in the orthopaedic ward for about six weeks. Every time the mother saw me in the ward or in the hospital corridor, she bent down to touch my feet and gave me lots of blessings. I told her that it was my duty, and she did not need to thank me so much.

Now, years later, when I think about this incident, I ask myself, "what made me go so much out of my way to help this boy." The only answer I can think of is that if Allah wants to do something, He will create the necessary circumstances. He has power over everything; He can make people work for Him.

It says in Surah Yusuf, *"Allah has overall power over all His affairs, but people know this not."* Surah: 12, Verse: 21. It was Allah who put thoughts in my mind to go out of my way to help this patient, as He put thoughts in Dr Nayak's mind to go out of his way to help me in preparation for my exams.

19. Baby brother

In 1984, I was working in Saudi Arabia. Once I had a ten-year-old Saudi boy admitted in the ICU. with horrific injuries to his chest and other parts of the body. He was involved in a car accident.

He was not doing very well, and his chances of survival were negligible.

While he was in the ICU., I noticed that his sister, who was in her early twenties, was there, next to her brother, all day, doing prayers and reading Quran. It was quite clear that her prayers were deeply sincere and intense. She did not lose hope even though the family was told about the bleak chances of the boy's survival. She continued her prayers and devotion.

Then we started seeing a positive change in the boy's condition. He kept improving and a few weeks later, he left the ICU.

Although I cannot prove scientifically, I still feel, even today, that her sister's prayers and devotion played a big role in his survival.

Can prayers change fate? I believe it can, but you still must do whatever is necessary; as in this case, we continued the treatment.

20. Power, pride, glory, respect, everything...available in market?

In 2005, in London, one of the imams, whom I knew very well, used to say this prayer regularly towards the end of Friday prayer's sermon: "Oh Allah, give back Muslims their power, pride, glory respect, etc., etc., which they had in the past."

However, he never said how to achieve them. Not even once, this imam or any imam in his sermon said how important worldly education is. How important the science and technology are? How important an industrial revolution is in Muslim countries. The reason is that they themselves do not realise the importance of these things. Most of our imams have only seen the religious schools in their lives. They are quite ignorant of the importance of science and technology. The imam who said to take out your brain if you want to follow Islam, also, in one of his sermons, said, "What have we got to do with the life cycle of mice? What have we got to do with channel four news and documentaries? He meant we, the Muslims, have nothing to do with any scientific experiment or with anything happening in the world. Then he continued his sermon, saying that we have come in this world to keep saying "Allah, Allah."

Once, I had a conversation with one of the worshipers. I told him about ISS (International Space Station) and Brexit. His response was, "We, Muslims, have nothing to do with these things." This approach is mainly due to a lack of understanding of Islam. In the past, there have been many Muslim scientists who have discovered/ invented many amazing things. For today's Muslims, Islam is confined to appearance and rituals. Other countries have gone sky high in science and technology. We always hear about China, India, and Brazil when it comes to industrial progress in the developing world. No Muslim country is included in this list.

Because of the wrong approach towards understanding Islam, the Muslim world is far behind the progressive world. Our imam prayed for Allah to give back Muslims, Power, Pride, Glory, etc.

Is power, pride, glory, and respect something available in the market? If so, I could have bought 10 kilos of power, 20 kilos of pride, 30 kilos of respect 40 kilos of glory and distributed it in the Muslim community.

Unless we understand Islam, put its principles into practice and excel in science, technology, industries, and agriculture, we are not going to get any of the above, i.e., power, respect, glory, pride, etc. Allah says in the Quran, *"We do not change the status of a nation unless the nation itself tries to do so"*, Surah: 13, verse: 11, surah: 8, verse: 53.

Friday's (22/12/2017) sermon in the same mosque. The imam was different.

He started moaning and groaning about Donald Trump, the US president, who had recently recognised Jerusalem as the capital of Israel. He went on to say how wrong and how unfair it was to do so. At the end, he asked the audience to pray that Donald Trump would reverse his decision and hand over Jerusalem to Muslims.

I did not pray, nor did I say Ameen at the end of his prayer because I knew that our prayers would not be answered. I have written the reasons above. The laws of nature (rules set up by God/Allah to run the world) do not change just because we pray and say Amin in a loud voice. See also chapter seven, "Allah is very kind to mankind," and chapter ten, "Who, Why, When, Where, How."

21. Preacher from the North-West Frontier

Once, I met a young man, in his 20s, in a mosque in Gillingham, Kent. He told me that he was from the North-West Frontier and was on a preaching tour of the UK. He gave me a talk on Islam and said everything which I already knew. I asked him what he did for a living. He said, "Nothing." He finished his religious course in his local religious school, never learnt a word of maths, science, and subjects like these. When he was living in his religious school, his teacher told him not to do any job and spend life "studying and preaching." I asked him how he met his expenses. He said that his brother bore all his expenses.

People who belong to this group go round, knocking on Muslims' doors, preaching to them everything which Muslims already know. When they came to my house, I told them that Islam is for everyone, why did they not go to my next-door neighbour, who was a Christian and preached him, Islam. The answer was, "first, we want to correct you." In their view, they are the only "correct" people who follow the true Islam and they want every Muslim to be like them.

Once upon a time, I was impressed by them and joined their group. I had been on a preaching tour in North West of England.

However, once I started listening to the book they read, I changed my mind and came out of their group. Their book has got so many flaws that it became unbearable for me to sit quietly and listen to it. When I raised objections, I was told to keep quiet as I was a junior member of the group; "How dare you challenge this book? It is written by famous, well-known scholars from India, do they know or do you know." There are many incidences/stories written in this book that are simply unbelievable and make Islam unworkable, impractical and without common sense.

Recently, a member of this group told me why they go round, preaching the same thing to Muslims only, what every Muslim already knows. He said that Coca-Cola is well known to everyone and yet it is advertised everywhere. He was trying to justify going from house to house of Muslims only and giving the same message again and again. I told him: "Coca-Cola is advertised for everyone. People of all faith see the advertisement. The advertisement is not for "Muslims only," so why do you not go to my next-door neighbour, a Christian, and give him the advertisement of Islam? The reason is that you cannot put a decent argument to promote your point of view." He did not say anything. When I was with this group, I realised that their knowledge of the Quran was very little. They give more importance to their book than to the Quran. They believe in everything written in this book. There are billions and billions of books in this world and yet the Quran is the only one that claims, *"No falsehood can come into it from the front or behind (any side) as it is sent down by One who has ultimate wisdom and is worthy of all praise"* Surah: 41, verse: 42.

Going by this, no book is perfect, and yet people who belong to this group believe in every single word written in this book.

However, I must admit that these people are very humble, meek, honest, and innocent. They are innocent to such an extent that they believe every single word of this book.

22. No pulse, no blood pressure

In the 1960s, in my second year of medical school, we had a lecture on the heart and blood vessels and pulse and blood pressure. The normal pulse rate is 72 beats a minute and normal blood pressure is 120/80.

A week later, the lecturer brought a Sadhu (Hindu priest) in the classroom and asked us to take his pulse rate and blood pressure. They were within the normal range. Then the lecturer said that the priest was going to make his pulse and blood pressure disappear.

The priest went into Trans, and ten minutes later, he was in a sleepy state. His pulse and blood pressure had disappeared. A few minutes later, he woke up and his pulse and blood pressure were back to normal. I do not know how he did it. Apparently, there are people who can train themselves to do so. Apparently, it is a matter of mind over matter.

The only scientific explanation is that these people train themselves to increase their vagal tone to a very high level. This reduces the heart rate to very low levels with undetected pulse and with this reduces the blood pressure as well.

Years later, in England, I have seen some trauma and some non-trauma cases with extremely low/non-existent pulse and blood pressure. One of my exam questions was how to differentiate between a deeply comatose patient and a dead person.

The mind over matter reminded me of one question my non-Muslim colleague once asked me. He asked: "In Scotland, in summer, fasting in the month of Ramadhan is for very long hours, almost 20 hours; how do you do this?" My answer was: "It is a matter of mind over matter."

23. Drag him...

No Muslim denies the importance of congregational prayers in the mosque. However, rules should be followed with some common sense. Following is written in a well-known religious book:

If a person is sick and cannot come to the mosque for the prayers by himself, then two people from the mosque should go to his house and "drag" him to the mosque, and after the prayer is finished, "drag" him back to his house. This should be repeated for every prayer, i.e., five times a day.

The book is written in the Urdu language, and the word used to bring the sick person to the mosque actually means "drag." It would have been better if the writer would have written that the people from the mosque should make some arrangement to bring the sick person to the mosque, for example, by car, if the sick person wishes to do so and if there is no risk to his health and life.

There is so much flexibility in the religion, but it needs common sense.

24. Obedience without common sense

A Muslim friend of mine was showing me his wedding photographs. In one photo, he was sitting on a chair and the bride was washing his feet with milk. I was astonished. This person was a regular worshiper in the local mosque and was a "practising" Muslim. I asked him why he agreed to such an act, i.e., using milk to wash his feet that too by the bride. His answer was, "what can I do? It was my mother's order."

There may be some occasions when we must disobey our parents. Examples are when Ibrahim (A.S.) disobeyed his father, and in Surah 31, verses 14 and 15.

44

Here Allah is asking you to treat your parents nicely and kindly and yet disobey them if they ask you to do something against the fundamentals.

25. Widow in a wedding

In some cultures, in India, a widow is not allowed to come anywhere near the bride. A widow is regarded as an "unlucky" woman (because her husband had died) and she would bring bad luck to the bride.

My wife told me that in my daughter's wedding, during a "women-only ceremony", a well-respected, religious woman, who teaches Quran as well, prevented my mother-in-law, a widow, from coming near my daughter because "widow is an unlucky" woman. This woman was lucky that I was not there.

After I heard this, I made sure that my mother-in-law was present in all other ceremonies and did what she was supposed to do.

Some people read the Quran, teach the Quran and yet their cultural and other believes dominate their views.

26. Six months later

It is a common belief that people in India, Pakistan and other developing countries are corrupt and cheats. Not all of them.

While working in Saudi Arabia, I went for Umrah (pilgrim to Mecca), by coach. While waiting at the coach station in Madinah, to come back to Dammam, a man approached me. He looked Pakistani. He told me that he was also there for Umrah and his wallet had been stolen. He needed to go back to Kuwait, where he was working. He wanted 700 Riyals from me. This sort of story is very common there and I had been warned about this.

First, I refused. The man turned away and started going back. The disappointment on his face was very touching. I called him back and gave him the money. He asked for my address in Dammam. I gave my address, but I was sure that I would not get my money back. He said he would return the money in two weeks' time.

I came back to Dammam. Two weeks had gone, then two months gad gone, there was no money in the post. I forgot all about it.

Six months later, I got a letter from him, with the money. He apologised for the delay and said when he reached Kuwait, he heard that his mother was very ill, so he had to go back to Lahore. This was the reason for the delay.

There are good Muslims.

27. It is 15 Rupees and not 25

While visiting Hyderabad, I went to a nearby mosque. There was a poster in the mosque hanging on the wall. It had sayings of Hazarat Ali (R.A), the 4th Khalif. I liked the poster and wanted some photocopies of it. There was a young boy, 15/16 years old, standing near me. He looked quite poor. I asked him if he could make some photocopies of the poster. He said yes. I told him to make five copies. He said it would be 25 rupees, i.e., 5 rupees/copy. I said OK and told him that I would come for the next prayer.

I met the boy during the next prayer. He gave me five copies of the poster and I gave him 25 rupees and started walking out of the mosque. The boy came running after me. He said the total cost was 15 rupees and he gave me back 10 rupees. I was very impressed by his honesty. Surely his parents must have brought him up very nicely.

On my next visit to the mosque, I gave him x amount of money as a gift.

There have been incidences like this in Pakistan, London and other places.

There are nice and honest people everywhere, Muslims and non-Muslims.

28. My words are...

When my sister retired in Hyderabad, she got a lump sum. She made a deal with a person to buy his flat in six lakhs (600,000) rupees. The man was known to her sons and was a regular worshiper in the local mosque. It was a verbal deal and to be in writing later.

It emerged that some other person approached the seller, and offered him a much higher price. The seller refused to accept the higher price saying that a deal had been done with my sister. The buyer said it was not in writing and, therefore, could be broken. The seller said: "My words are as good as a written deal."

All such people are God-fearing and keep the "hereafter" in their minds.

29. What can I do, doctor...I am not allowed...

An Asian Muslim lady in her 40s came for a mastectomy operation (removal of the breast due to cancer).

When she arrived in the operation theatres, her top clothes were removed by the nurses to gain access for surgery and also to put various monitors like an ECG.

As the clothes were removed, her armpits were stinking with the smell of sweat. The smell spread in the operation theatres quickly and everyone was feeling it. I asked the lady in her language (Urdu/Panjabi) as to why she had not put some deodorant in her armpits before coming to theatres. Her answer was: "what can I do doctor, in my religion, i.e., Islam, ladies are not allowed to put on any perfume."

Comments: Rules should be followed with common sense. In this case, the interpretation was totally wrong. There is absolutely no common sense in this. What is discouraged is the ladies wearing too much perfume and going around attracting the attention of men. This is for their own safety.

This is just one of the many miss-interpretations of rules and regulation which are meant to give moral laws and create a clean society. I cannot blame this lady because she followed what was told to her by her husband or other men of the house and I cannot blame the men either because they followed what they read or were told by the religious leaders in the local mosques.

There are many examples of misinterpretations of verses of the Quran and other rules and regulations. For example Surah: 4, Verse: 34. The translation of this verse in Asian Qurans is "Man is the master and woman is a slave", while the translation in Arab Quran is "Man is the breadwinner and protector of woman."

30. Sorry, but I have only one wife

I read this story in a religious book which I found in a London mosque.

Person A (the host) was a very pious and religious person. He had a friend, B, (the guest) who lived in another place, and he was also a very pious and religious person.

B, the guest, wrote to his friend A, the host, that he was coming to his place and was going to stay with him for few weeks.

When the guest arrived, the host had made all the arrangements for his comforts. He showed the guest his room and everything there. Then the host said to the guest: "I am very sorry, I have only one wife. If I had two wives, I would have given you one."

Comments: Is a woman a "thing" to be used by anyone? Does she not have her own free will? Does she not have her own liking and disliking, her feelings, her emotions? Is she supposed to be an obedient wife and sleep with another man, like it or not?

Is this Islamic literature? Is the writer of this book a scholar?

31. By God, I have no money

My brother was working in the Abu Dhabi air force. He told me the following true story: He (my brother) was in his office. His friend Abdul, from Pakistan, was with him as well. Abdul belonged to a particular "preaching party." They go round to Muslim houses only, preaching the same thing which every Muslim knows.

The pay clerk walked into the office and gave Abdul his monthly salary, in cash, which was a few thousand Dirhams. Abdul kept this cash in the top pocket of his shirt. A few minutes later, Abdul's friend, Malik, came into the office and asked Abdul if he could lend him some money. Abdul put his hand on the right hip pocket and said to Malik: "I swear by Allah, I have no money." Malik was disappointed and went away. My brother asked Abdul why he said he had no money and that too, swearing by Allah when he had thousands of Dirhams in his shirt pocket.

Abdul said: "the pocket, on which I put my hand and swore by Allah, was my hip pocket and it had no money. The money is in my shirt pocket, not in my hip pocket."

Comments: Wonderful excuse to justify his actions. The Quran, in many places, says that if you cannot afford to lend, say some nice and comforting words, politely and nicely.

This person was a preacher of Islam.

32. "Do not give women their share."... *Really?*

Some time ago, I was in a mosque for the mid-day prayer. After the prayer, there was a session of the teaching and explanation of the Quran. I stayed to attend this session. Going through the beginning of the 4th Surah, the teacher, who was also the imam of the mosque, when it came to the 5th verse, said something which I found extremely displeasing.

In this verse, Allah is saying not to give the rightful share of the inheritance to that those who are weak in understanding. The word used is "suffuha." Here, "those who are weak in understanding" means children whose parents have died and they are not yet old enough to understand and manage their share of the inheritance. The verse continues to say that the trustee should treat them nicely and give them the inheritance once they can manage it.

The imam said that the word "suffuha" has two meanings, 1. Children who are too young to understand the money matters. 2. Women.

His first meaning was right, but explaining the 2nd meaning, he said that women are silly, stupid, spendthrift, careless, etc., etc. Therefore, they should not get their share of the inheritance. Here, he is one million per cent wrong. The verse does not mean this at all, no other imam has said this, and I did not find this explanation in any other book. This is probably, this imam's personal view.

However, imams are well respected by the Muslim community. The general Muslim population believes in them and anything they say. This imam has spent seven years studying religion in a well-known religious school in India. Where did he get this kind of thinking from? I have come across such religious people who say that women should be kept at the tip of their shoes. This is one million per cent un-Islamic thinking. Have they not read in the Quran how much respect Maryam (Mary, A.S.), mother of Jesus (A.S.) and the Pharos's wife is given? How respectful were Khudiaja, Ayesha, Fatima (R.A.) and many other Muslim women?

Even at an ordinary level, there are some very good Muslim women and very bad Muslim men. My eldest sister became a widow at a time when her children were young. She brought them up very nicely, educated them very well and gave them very good, sensible religious education as well. By the grace of Allah, all of them are very well off. I am sure there are many examples like this.

Unfortunately, even here in the UK, there are people who believe in the above-mentioned imam and in religious people like him.

No wonder why you go to any Sharia council; the maximum number of complaints are from women against their husbands or against their brothers. Husbands are not treating them well and brothers are not giving them their share of the inheritance. There are so many verses in the Quran which says to treat women nicely and give them their fair share but below I am writing what the Prophet (PBUH) said in his last sermon:

"O people, it is true that you have certain rights with regard to your women, but they also have rights over you. If they abide by your rights, then to them belongs the right to be fed and clothed in **kindness**. Do treat your women well and be kind to them, for they are your partners and committed helpers."

Further down the sermon, the Prophet is reminding us, "Remember, one day you will meet your Lord and give the account of your deeds".

33. Very sensible

Tuesday 30 May 2017. (4th Ramadhan 1438H). 8:50 p.m.

After the prayer, in my local mosque, London E11, there was a speech by a Mufti from the Stamford Hill Mosque, London.

His topic was–being content and not being greedy and how to achieve a balance between the two.

I appreciated him very much. He spoke very nicely and sensibly, without any controversial points. We need people like him. He seemed to be aware of current affairs and said things that attract and meet the needs of young people.

I could add few points to his speech because I have also thought about this topic. The reason for my thinking was, in the same mosque, some time ago, another imam, in his speech, said: *"do a normal job, but do not do overtime."* I disagreed with him.

Then one of my doctor friends phoned me and said that the hospital was short of staff and asked him to do an overtime shift. My friend was in two minds. He thought, by doing an overtime shift, he was being greedy and not content with what he has got.

I explained to him that Allah does not forbid a man to make his living better and better and have a comfortable life. The important thing is that you do not violate the fundamental principles of Islam and do not ignore the rights to Allah, rights to yourself and rights to others, and in this case, the rights to your family.

I told him to ask some questions to himself: 'If I do this over time, will I miss my five daily prayers? If it is Ramadhan, will I miss my fasting? Am I ignoring my wife and my children? Am I putting my health and wellbeing in danger by doing this overtime? If the answer to any of these questions is yes, then do not do the overtime.'

There were many companions of the Prophet (PBUH) who were very rich and had big businesses. Examples are Abu-Bakar, Usman, Abu Ayyub Ansari (R.A.) The Prophet never asked them to wind down their business. We have a very good example in them. They earned more but:

a. It was all Halal (legal) money earned via legal means.
b. They were never proud of it.
c. They never showed off their wealth.
d. They did not violate any principle of Islam or ignored their rights to Allah, rights to themselves, or rights to their families or other human beings.
e. They never looked down upon others who were less well off than them.
f. They spent their wealth for the right purpose, to please Allah, in serving humanity.
g. They did not compete with others. They were content with their efforts and what Allah had given to them.

In other words, *hereafter* was always in their mind.

If one can do all the above, then there is no harm in earning more.

34. Can you believe it?

a) In the 1950s, 60s, 70s, and probably even now, in the Indian subcontinent, especially in the villages, the treatment of any illness was not by medicines but by village saints and those who could perform an exorcism. All illnesses were supposed to be due to some spirit possessing the patient.

However, just yesterday, 13/06/2017, it was in the news that in Oregon, USA, a young couple, devote Christians, refused to let their sick, three-month-old baby have any modern treatment. They opted for "faith healing." It did not work, and the baby died.

In the 21st century, in the most advanced country in the world, do we still have people like the above couple?

42) Jealousy has an effect-take one:

It was a Sunday evening; I was at my home when a lady and her grown-up son came to visit us. As we were chatting, the son started complaining about his boss at work, as to how bad he was, how strict he was, how short-tempered he was, etc.

Then the lady asked me how my boss was? I told her that I did not have a boss.

Consultants do not have any bosses; they are independent practitioners. The lady's face suddenly changed, and she gave me such a "jealous look" that I felt her piercing eyes. I felt very uneasy with her look. She was comparing me with her son. That night I could not sleep. The lady's jealous face and her piercing eyes kept coming back as flashes in my mind.

The next day was Monday. As usual, I was in the hospital at 7:30 a.m. Around 9 a.m., the managers came to the operation theatres, took me to a corner and said that there had been complaints against me regarding the treatment I was providing and the complications the patients were developing. He said that they were investing those complaints and until they were fully investigated, I could not work independently. I needed permission and supervision from my colleagues. I was very shocked to hear that. Now, suddenly, overnight, *I had bosses* to answer. They were my colleagues and my juniors. Some of them were juniors. Even they were feeling very bad to supervise me. Five days passed. I had to seek permission from my junior colleagues to do every case; I had to show them my treatment and management plan and had to accept their advice. Those five days were extremely demoralising and depressing for me. At the end of the working week, i.e., Friday, around 4 p.m., the managers came to the operation theatres and told me that they had fully investigated the complaints against me and could not find any fault in my work and I was free to work independently.

Jealousy does hurt you but only as much as Allah has written in your fate; (Quran).

42) Jealously has an effect take two:

The hospital was short of staff, so the secretary asked me if I could do some extra work. I said OK. After finishing the extra work over the weekend, on Monday, I took the papers to the secretary so that she could process them for the payment. The claim was for X amount. She looked at the papers and said: "Oh my God! What you have earned in two days, I don't earn this much in a month." The jealousy was very clear on her face.

I came back home. The next morning when I came out to go to the hospital, I found that my car had been vandalised. I had to take it to the garage. I informed the hospital that I was going to be late. As I was driving to the garage, smoke started coming out of the engine. I called the AA. They towed the car to the garage. In two days' time, the garage repaired the car. The bill was for X amount, the same as what I had earned by doing the extra work.

All good and harm ultimately come from Allah. In this, there is a test for us; (Quran).

35. Two extremes

I was in the operation theatres in a London hospital when the sister from the ward called me to come and see two patients who were due to have surgery on that day but had come late. Normally, I see all my patients before I go to the operation theatres so that I would not be disturbed in my work in the theatres. I was not very happy with the latecomers. However, I left my junior (experienced and trustable) to carry on in the theatres and went to the ward. The sister pointed me towards two beds where the new arrivals were. On the first bed, there was no patient, but there was a small tent-like structure in the middle of the bed. I asked the sister what that was. She told me that there is a female patient inside the tent. She was a Muslim lady from one of the Asian countries. She did not speak a single word of English and did not allow even the shadow of any man anywhere near her. The sister told me that with great difficulty, nurses managed to take her pulse and blood pressure. Her son was there as an interpreter, but he himself spoke very little English. I told the sister that I must see her, talk to her and examine her before she could come to the theatres for surgery; otherwise the operation would be cancelled. When the manager heard this, he came running and asked me if I could find a lady colleague of mine to see this patient and deal with her. I went back to the theatres, talked to one of my English lady colleagues who agreed to deal with this patient.

Then I went to see the 2nd patient. This was a 23-year-old girl. Her father was sitting in a chair about three feet from her. The girl was asthmatic, and her chest did not sound good. I took a nurse with me and told her that I needed to examine her in more detail, and she needed to take her top off completely. Then I turned round to her father and asked her to go out because her daughter was going to take her top off, including her bra. The father said: "It doesn't matter," and the girl nodded her head in agreement. Now she was completely naked from the waist above, not even the bra and her father was looking at her, just three feet from her.

What a contrast! In the next bed, there was a woman in the "tent."

Is this not two extremes? Right and wrong of this? I will leave the reader to decide.

I have no intention to criticise anyone's values, cultures, etc. I am writing this because all the staff found it "Strange but True."

36. Five different news and one definite conclusion

News number one: 30 May 2017. NASA (National Aeronautics and Space Agency) of the United States decided to send a probe to the sun of our solar system to study the solar wind and flares. These affect the weather and communication systems on earth. The probe will go as close as four million miles from the surface of the sun. This will happen in mid-2018.

News number two: 30 May 2017. The United States has successfully tested its "anti-missile defence system". A missile was blasted from point A and it was deducted, intercepted and destroyed by the system.

News number three: 31 May 2017. Russia has blasted five hypersonic missiles, 5-6 times the speed of sound.

News number four: 30 May 2017. A big car bomb blasted in Kabul, Afghanistan, killing 90 people and injuring 350 people. This was done in Ramadhan 1438 H. Muslims killed Muslims in Ramadhan.

News number five: 03/06/ 2017. Carnage at London Bridge. I feel so sorry for the victims and their families. Unfortunately, it was Muslims who were responsible for this, that too in the month of Ramadhan. Are they really Muslims? Do they really understand Islam? We, the Muslims in the UK, should be loyal to this country and do everything possible for its prosperity and peace. The fairness and justice you find here you will not find in your own country.

Conclusion: Who deserves to rule the world? The conclusion is very clear; it is not rocket science.

37. Seven earths

31 May 2017. NASA has discovered seven earth like planets in a solar system, 40 light-years (235 trillion miles) away from our solar system.

The Quran says in chapter 65, last verse: "It is Allah Who has made seven skies (heavens) and earth of a similar number…"

38. Coincidences are Allah's will

A) From "four hours" to "twenty-seven years."

In the early 1980s, I was working in Dumfries, Scotland. It was a very good town, and I had a very good job. However, we were missing London. So, I decided to leave that job and come back to London and try and find a job here, in London.

In London, I did not have a regular job. I was doing agency work. This job was on a day-to-day basis, depending on the needs of the hospitals nearby. If you work on a day, you are paid for that day only. In today's term (year 2017), it was Zero hours contract. On some days, I did not get any work. The income was irregular and the four essentials in a job were not there, i.e., a) permanent contract, also known as a substantive contract or open-ended contract. B) Paid annual leave, c) paid sick leave and d) pension contributions. If I fell ill, I was not paid, if I go on holiday, I was not paid, and I was not saving for my pension. Had I died, my young family would have been left penniless. I was not happy with the situation, but I had to carry on as I had two young children and a wife to support as well. All the time, I was praying to come out of this situation.

One day the agency sent me to a hospital in East London, to work for only four hours: 9 a.m. to 1 p.m. This was the only work on that day, after a gap of few days.

I finished my work at 1 p.m. and went to the changing room of the operation theatres to change and go to the secretary's office to get my papers signed for the payment. As I was changing, "A" man walked into the changing room and asked me: "For how long you are here for; Dr Khan?" I told him that I was there for four hours only. He looked at me for few seconds and then these words came out of his mouth: "You will never leave this place." I did not know who he was; I had never met him in my life (later, he turned out to be the theatre manager and had nothing to do with my agency or any power to give me more work in the hospital). He just said that one sentence and walked out of the changing room.

I went to the secretary's office to have the papers signed for the four hours of work payment. She asked me, "Are you free tomorrow?" I said yes and she offered me one full day's work next day. The next day she offered me more work and so on. Two weeks later, the head of the department came and asked me if I was happy to take a permanent post in that hospital. I was overjoyed. My prayers had been answered.

The hospital where I went to work for four hours as a consultant, I stayed there for 27 years. Those 27 years were the best years of my life. I was well established in my job. I was very popular in the hospital; I was well respected and well-liked. I actively took part in educational activities (my favourite hobby). However, I had some colleagues who were very jealous of me, who tried their best to get rid of me. By the grace of God, each time they tried, each time they failed. It is sad to say that these people were from my own place, i.e., the Indian subcontinent.

Overall, my time in that hospital was very good and I can only say that Allah had sent that theatre manager to the changing room and put those words in his mouth to relieve my anxiety about not having a regular job.

B) Pathology exam: In the 1960s, I was a medical student. Pathology is a difficult subject. Our book "Boyd's pathology" had over 1500 pages.

I had studied but did not pay much attention to diseases not common in India. Pernicious anaemia was one of them.

On the day of the exam, while travelling in public transport, I decided to have a look at "anything" in my notes. I randomly opened my notes; the topic was "Pernicious anaemia." I read the few pages, assuring myself that this would not be asked. I had not seen a single case of Pernicious anaemia in my life.

In the exam hall, the question paper was handed over and the first question was: "Write an essay on Pernicious anaemia."

C) Anatomy exam: Anatomy of the entire body, except the Brain, was in the curriculum for the first two years of medical studies. I did study but got "lost" in the human brain. I spent a lot of time studying the human brain. This made me weak in the anatomy of the rest of the body. While studying the brain, I had studied the anatomy of "Head and neck." I was very confident about it.

In the exam hall, I was given a limb and abdomen. Two examiners came along, asked me questions on these two specimens. I did not do well and knew that I had failed. The examiners started walking back to their table. I looked up and said in my mind: "Oh. God, please…After going about twenty steps, the examiners came back. There was a head and neck lying on the table. They asked me ten questions. I gave brilliant answers, extending into the "Brain" They were very pleased. I passed.

For others, it may look like a coincidence, but even today (2021), I believe God had answered my prayer, put the thought in the examiners' minds, and they came back.

It is just like the **"Hand of God",** mentioned by Diego Maradona, the Argentinian footballer, who made the winning goal against England in the 1986, FIFA quarter-final.

I am sure these sorts of coincidences happen with other people as well.

I believe that Allah (God, or whatever you call and believe) can put thoughts in a person's mind which either help him or harm him. Here are a few more coincidences I remember from the news:

A. A man planned a family holiday abroad. He, his wife and three children arrived at the airport. At the last moment, the man got a call related to his work. He told his wife and children to board the flight, and he would take the next flight after sorting out the work-related issue. The family took the flight without him, and the plane crashed. All the family members died.

B. The T.W.A. flight from Toronto to Delhi was brought down by a bomb over Southern Ireland. A Sikh man was supposed to board that flight, but at the Toronto airport, he got so lost in the duty-free shop that he missed the flight. This saved his life.

C. A lady was killed in the disaster in a football stadium. She was least interested in football, had never been to a football match. She was given a ticket by her friend to see the match.

D. When I was in India, I heard of so many incidences where people either missed or boarded a train and this either saved or killed them.

Here are some verses from Quran:

1. Allah (God) has power over everything. Surah 2, Verses 20 and 284, Surah 11, verse number 4 and many more.

2. Allah (God) has full control over His affairs, but many of the men do not know this. Surah 12, verse 21.

3. There is not a single creature on the earth whose ultimate control is not in God's hand. Surah 11, verse 56. (a phrase is used in this verse which means ultimate control).

4. No matter what you wish, what happens ultimately is what Allah wishes. Surah 81, last verse.

5. There are so many verses that end in sentences like, Allah knows, and you do not. Allah is all Knower, all Wise.

39. Museum of failure: (BBC news, 8 June 2017)

Samuel West is a psychologist in Sweden. He has opened a museum named "Museum of failure". He has collected all the new inventions and products which were developed by various scientists and inventors but failed to materialise in everyday life. As a psychologist, he wants to show that there is "success" in "failure."

I always believed that failures could lead to success if: a) you learn from your failures and correct yourself; b) do not give up, do not get disheartened.

There are many examples in history, but the best is the "Treaty of Hudaibia" in Islamic history. In this, there was an apparent failure with humiliation. The Prophet and his companions were prevented from entering Mecca. However, the way the Prophet dealt with it was amazing and showed his farsightedness. It also showed how loyal the companions were to him. This *apparent failure* ultimately led to the success of the conquest of Mecca without any bloodshed. The temporary defeats (failures) in the battles of Uhad and Hunain, which ultimately turned into victory (success), are other examples of wisdom, courage, perseverance, learning from the failures and not giving up. In the Quran, in many places, Allah asks us to stay steadfast and not lose hope: Surah 12, verse 87, Surah 31, verse 17, and many more.

When Apollo 13 and Apollo 11 missions ended in disaster, NASA did not give up. It analysed the reasons for failures, corrected itself and moved on.

When the late Mrs Margaret Thatcher did her graduation, she applied for a job in the ICI (Imperial Chemical Industries). She failed to get a job. She did not give up and ultimately became the Prime Minister of the United Kingdom.

Even at an ordinary level, there are so many men and women who turn their failures into success. However, some do not and either give up or even commit suicide.

The psychology of failure and how to deal with it is a big chapter. The important thing is not to give up, learn from the failure and not lose hope. This is the teaching in all religions.

40. Friday, 9 June 2017 (14th Ramadhan 1438 H)

On the above day, I went to the local mosque for the Friday prayer. I arrived about 40 minutes early. The speaker for the sermon was somebody from India. When he came and sat on the pulpit, I said to myself, "OMG, why did I come early." The speaker looked very uneducated, unimpressive, typical mullah-type person, somebody who had been dragged from some remote village of India. I had no choice but to stay because the Friday prayer was after his sermon. I was not expecting anything worthwhile from this person.

However, when he started speaking, it was so nice and impressive that I listened to the whole sermon attentively. He did not say a silly thing. He was referring to the Quran and Sunnah all the time and spoke about an Islam, which was workable and practical in the western world, an Islam in which there is NO place for terrorism.

This speaker was also from a famous religious school in India. I have listened to the other speakers from the same school. They talk a mixture of nice, good things and a silly, unbelievable, impractical Islam. They cannot differentiate between what is right and what is silly.

There are two questions I have been thinking about for years and still cannot find satisfactory answers: a) why two persons qualified from the same religious school have such widely different views that one person says nothing but nice and sensible things while the other says all silly things?

42) People who have never been to any religious school acquire, by self-study, such good and sensible knowledge about the religion that they are far better than those who had been to the religious school; How?

I have worked out the answers to the above questions, which, in my view, are closest to the right answers, but I will leave the reader to make up his/her own mind.

41. Mujahid-e-Islam (Jihadist)

In my local mosque, it was announced that a mujtahid (one who fights an Islamic battle) was coming to give a speech about jihad. This fighter, apparently, had taken part in battles against the invaders in an Asian country.

I went to listen to his speech. He started by saying some historical battles in the early days of Islam. This was history and was common knowledge. There was nothing new for me in it. Then he said the following in connection with his own battlefield:

He was fighting on the battlefield, along with his other fighter colleagues. The battle started in the morning and went on all day. One of his colleague fighters, a young man, was shot and killed by enemy fire.

In the evening, at the end of the fight, he and his friends wanted to bury the young man who had died. As they dug the grave and were about to put the body in the grave, our fighter speaker told his people to wait and inform the father of the dead young man, in case the father wanted to come and say goodbye to his son. Somebody ran to the young man's house and informed the father. The father said he wanted to come and attend the burial. When the father came to the battleground and saw his son's dead body, he addressed the dead body and said, "if you are a real martyr, get up now and tell me." The dead man came back to life, got up and told his father that he was a real martyr and then dropped dead.

It was noticeably clear that this speaker, one who has fought in the path of Allah, was saying nothing but lies. Then the speaker narrated this verse from Quran, Surah 2, and verse 154: *"Those who are killed in the path of Allah do not call them dead, they are alive."* Then the speaker said that this verse was proof that the young man was a martyr. For his own gain, he mentioned an incomplete verse. The full verse is like this:" *Those who are killed in the path of Allah, do not call them dead, they are alive, but you perceive it not."*

Standing in the mosque, as a well-respected speaker, he said such a big lie. He purposely narrated an incomplete verse from the Quran just to prove his point. God only knows how many fighters are like this who are quite happy to tell lies. I am glad that they do not get any victory. If they are victorious, what kind of Islamic government would they establish in the land? Would everything be according to the Quran and Sunnah but twisted and distorted to suit their needs and their views?

At the end of his speech, I wanted to ask him about this whole saga, especially the fact that he mentioned an incomplete verse from the Quran, just to prove his point which itself was a lie. As usual, he was surrounded by people who were very impressed by him. These were his devotees, the blind believers.

It is very easy to fool people in the name of the religion, especially the Muslims.

42. Even sky is not the limit

This world and its amenities and facilities are available to all of us. It is up to the individuals how to use them. For this, even the sky is not the limit.

The best examples of doing nothing but good are the lives of all the messengers of God in every religion. Religious books have many examples of people who did nothing but bad, e.g., The Pharos.

Even in today's world, there are so many opportunities to do right/ wrong. Right and wrong are relative terms. Many "wrongs" in the 1940/50s are right in

2021. My memories date back to 1954. Some of the things I have written in this book need to be taken with that context of time, i.e., the 1950s/60s in India.

I had some interesting experiences in my life. Here are few examples:

a) I was flying back from Hyderabad to London via Bombay. I stayed in a hotel in Bombay, near the airport, for the night.

I was in my room, had just finished the night prayer, around 9 p.m. I was still sitting on the prying mattress; there was a knock on the door. When I opened the door, there was a hotel worker standing at the door. He asked me, "Do you want a girl for the night?" and before I said 'No', he went on to describe the varieties of the girls he had and their special features. He described them like a menu in a restaurant.

My answer was, of course, 'No'.

I feel sorry for the girls who end up like this.

Apparently, prostitution is the oldest "profession" in the world.

b) After the mid-day prayer, I was coming out of the local mosque in London. I saw another person, JB, whom I knew well, coming out of the mosque as well. He looked very angry. I asked him what the matter was, then jokingly said to him: "If your wife has told you off, it is nothing new, it is our (men's) fate, we are in it together, are you not used to it by now?". He did not smile at my joke and said: "Do you have any house for sale near your home?" I asked him why he wanted to move. He said that the prostitution had increased so much in the area where he lived that the girls and ladies from the nice families, who return from their universities and work in the evening, are taken as prostitutes and approached by the clients.

If you go to that area after sunset, you will get all kinds of offers and temptations, including buy one, get another half price.

c) One Friday late night, I was coming back from Heathrow airport after dropping a visitor. Normally I take the M25 or A406 route. This time I thought it was a late-night, there should not be much rush, and I should take the central London route, which comes via King's Cross. As I was

61

at Kings Cross, for some reason, there was a traffic jam. I had no choice but to wait. Then the prostitutes started banging my window: "Sir, you want to have some fun? Sir, have you tried three in a bed? It is really fun; for me, it is £25, for my friend, pay half price, we will come to your place, or you come to ours. The back of the car seat is just £5 and only one go". I kept saying in my mind: "I seek refuge in Allah from the Shaitan (devil), the rejected." My prayers were answered, and the traffic moved.

d) A French lady doctor used to work with me. She was unmarried and lonely. She made many passes on me. Once, she told me: "I know you are married, but there is no harm in having a bit of fun…"

43. You wear a tie

On some occasions, I went to the mosque on my way back from the hospital. Obviously, I used to be in western clothes, a suit and tie or jacket, trousers and a tie.

On one such occasion, the Imam again repeated that women are not allowed in the mosque, and he gave the usual explanation that at the time of Umar (R.A.), the second Khalif, women were becoming too liberal, so he consulted with Ayesha (R.A.) and between them, they decided to ban women from coming to the mosque.

I put my points to him in favour of allowing women to come to mosques. At the top of my points was that women are human beings, and they should be treated with dignity and respect. My other points were some verses from the Quran, some points from the Sunnah and common sense.

The Imam's reply was: 'a) Why should I/we listen to you? You do not have a certificate from any religious school. b) You work with non-Muslims and are influenced by them and their culture. c) You are westernised. d) You wear western clothes. e) You wear a tie, and a tie is the symbol of the cross. You walk into the mosque with the cross in your neck. If I have power, I will ban anyone entering "**my**" mosque who wears a tie.'

The only thing I could think at that time in my mind was, "God save us from such imams and their Islam."

This imam was not the only one: on another occasion, some other religious person told me in the same mosque that if he had power, he would demolish all the Muslim houses which have TVs. What he did not know that people walk around with their mobile phones, even in the mosque. On mobile phones, you can watch everything which you can watch on TV.

My advice to him was: Kill the desire to watch wrong things rather than kill the TV, mobile phones, computers, iPad, etc.

44. Weekend wife

In every big organisation, including hospitals, there is a procurement department, and all the purchases will have to be approved by it. Usually, there is a committee consisting of representatives from each department who decide what to buy.

I was the representative on this committee from my department. Usually, there is an unwritten rule that all the members support each other's recommendations for purchases. For example, if an orthopaedic surgeon wants to buy a particular instrument for his department, and he chooses one particular brand from many, the other members do not object to that (mainly because they do not know much about that instrument). Medical representatives come to these meetings as well, bring their company's products, and persuade (even gently bribe) the potential buyer (a doctor from a particular department) to recommend to the hospital to buy their product.

On one such occasion, a gynaecologist, Mr R, was being persuaded by the medical representative to buy his company's product. The following conversation took place between them:

Medical rep to Mr R: "If you recommend to the hospital to buy our company's product, our company will send you and your wife to Paris for a weekend, you will stay in a five-star hotel and you will have a chauffeur-driven car to go round Paris."

Mr R to the medical rep: "I will go to Paris, but not with my wife. Only a fool will go to Paris with his wife."

Medical rep to Mr R: "Don't worry, Doc, we will supply you a weekend wife."

When the other doctors in the committee objected to this, they said that they were joking. I do not think they were joking.

45. Right patient, wrong procedure...importance of communication

There have been cases in the hospitals where wrong procedures/operations were done on patients, for example, amputation of the right leg instead of left leg, removal of right kidney instead of left kidney, etc. The common factors among such mistakes are: a) Miscommunication. b) No attention to detail. c) Human error. d)The patients are asleep (General Anaesthesia), therefore cannot tell the doctors that he is operating on the wrong side. e) Medical staff under pressure/stress to finish the operating list on time.

However, I had a patient who was awake, had the wrong procedure done and yet did not say anything. The details are as follows:

I was making a gynaecology operating list. There were four patients on the list. Their anaesthetics were planned as follows:

1. First patient...General Anaesthetics.
2. Second patient...Spinal Anaesthetics.
3. Third patient...General Anaesthetics.
4. Fourth patient...General Anaesthetics.

We started the list with the first patient. During the operation, the gynaecologist and the nurse in charge were whispering and decided to do the fourth patient as next but did not tell me (I came to know about this later on).

As we were finishing the first patient, I asked the sister in charge to send for the next patient, assuming that she would send for one who was second in the list, who was supposed to have the spinal anaesthesia. She sent for number 4 (who was supposed to have general anaesthetics) but did not tell me.

When the next patient (No 4) arrived in the anaesthetic room, thinking that it was patient No 2, I asked my registrar to go and put the spinal anaesthesia in her (she was supposed to have general anaesthesia). The registrar had not seen the patient beforehand, so he did not recognise that the patient was to have general anaesthesia and not the spinal.

He put the spinal anaesthesia.

The mistake was recognised when I saw the patient in the operation theatre. She was fully awake and asked me: "When am I going to sleep?"

Everyone was worried. I was the ultimately responsible consultant anaesthetist. I asked the sister in charge for the mistake. Her answer was: "Oh! I thought you heard our conversation about the change of the order of the list."

Duty of Candour: I explained to the patient the mistake and apologised. She was happy that I was honest and open.

Question: Does this patient carry any responsibility for the mistake? She was awake when the spinal analgesia was done and yet did not raise any concern as to "why are you giving me an injection in my back? when I am supposed to go to sleep?"

I presented this case in the "Grand Rounds" of the hospital, where over 50 doctors of all grades were present. The answer to this question from the majority of the doctors was: "The final responsibility of any mistake lies with the doctor."

In this case, I am not sure of the answer. Doctors are humans and can make mistakes. An awake patient has some responsibility towards the surgery he/she is having.

If you are having a cataract operation, under local anaesthetics, in your right eye and the surgeon starts putting local anaesthetics in your left eye, will you not ask why he is putting local anaesthetics in the left eye when the operation is to be done on the right eye? You are fully awake; therefore, you should ask.

Another non-medical incidence of miss communication.

This happened quite a few years ago, over Asia. I read it in the newspaper.

Plane A was going to country B. At the same time plane B was going to country A. As plane A was approaching country B, plane B had just taken off from country B. The two planes were going to cross each other's paths at dangerously close distance. The ground control from country B told plane A to descend down 400 feet. Not understanding correctly, the plane descended 400 meters. The result was a big bang with the loss of life in both planes.

The incidence is true, although the figures of distances and some other details may not be accurate as I am writing this with my memory.

Morel of the stories: Communicate loud and clear, especially if you are dealing with life.

46. £5

In a London hospital, I was called to the A & E to see a severely injured young man, about 18 years old.

In the A & E, the Asian boy was lying on the trolley. He was awake but was severely injured. My team and I started to do what was necessary. The mother of the boy was standing at the foot end of the trolley. As I was the senior-most person there, the junior staff was asking me for various instructions. Seeing that I was the consultant and an Asian, the mother of the boy called me in a corner and offered me £ 5 and said: "Doctor Sahib, please keep this money but take good care of my son." Of course, I did not take the money but assured her that we would (and we did) take good care of the injured boy. A few weeks later, he left the hospital on his feet.

Culture of Bribery: The point I want to make here is that in Asian countries, bribery is 'the' norm. I have seen this as a junior doctor doing my house job in India.

However, when the Asians come here to the western world, they still carry the same culture applicable to the Asians only. This woman would not have offered £5 if the consultant would have been an English man or anyone else but an Asian. She straight away assumed that being an Asian, I would take that £5 and, in return, would care for her son. They cannot imagine an environment free of bribery.

When my father retired in India in the 1950s, it took him one year to have his pension started because he refused to bribe the officials who were supposed to sort out his paperwork. Q: How do we educate our people?

(This is in sharp contrast to when I retired from the NHS. All my papers were sorted out well before my retirement date. I did not have to pay a single penny.)

47. "I can't do it; it is haram (forbidden)."

In a London hospital, I had a junior Muslim doctor with me who was new to the country.

I received a call from the A & E that the ambulance was bringing a young woman who was critically ill, and we (my junior and I) needed to be in the resuscitation room ASAP.

As we both went to the resuscitation room, I saw the woman being wheeled in. It was clear to me that she was unconscious and very ill. Other A & E doctors

66

were there. One was taking the history from the ambulance crew, while the others were preparing the "essentials."

I told my junior that we needed to put the monitors (ECG and others) and be ready to start CPR (Cardiopulmonary Resuscitation/ chest compression and artificial breathing). The woman was wearing a blouse and skirt. To put the ECG and defibrillator pads, we needed to cut the blouse and attach the ECG leads.

A pair of scissors was available, and I told my junior to cut the woman's blouse. He walked away. It was an "Every second counts" situation, so I did everything, including the chest compressions, etc. My junior came back and was watching me doing the chest compression. I told him to take over from me (chest compression is a back-breaking, exhaustive manoeuvre). He walked away.

Fortunately, the woman's circulation and heartbeat came back, and we shifted her to the ICU.

Later, I asked my junior to explain his behaviour. His answer was:

"I am forbidden by Islam to touch a strange woman who is "Non-mahram" * to me, let alone cut her blouse and do the chest compression."

I gave him a long lecture on understanding the underlying principle/s behind any rule and used common sense rather than reading/ listening about the rule and following it blindly. I told him that while world religions give guidelines on how to behave with the opposite sex, they are for social occasions, not for emergencies like these.

I warned him that any more behaviour like this, I would report to the managers and to the head of the department and he would be sacked.

Fortunately, such incidences are rare.

*A non-mahram is a person of the opposite sex who is marriageable to you, but not married to you.

A mahram is a person whom you cannot marry, e.g., mother, sister, aunt, uncle, etc.

Chapter Two
Whose Monopoly is Islam?

A mosque in London, E11, was to have an extension and to have the first floor built. In this mosque, ladies are not allowed. To raise funds for the building work, there was a meeting of management and the people who use the mosque. I was invited, so I attended the meeting and said that I was happy to contribute, but once the building work was done, we should have more capacity and therefore, ladies should be allowed in the mosque. The president of the mosque committee and other members agreed. The work started and finished after few months. There was an inauguration ceremony. I was hoping that it would be announced that since now we had a bigger mosque, a portion of it would be for the ladies to pray. Instead, the main Imam stood up and gave a speech saying that ladies were not allowed in this or any mosque. He gave a historical reason saying that at the time of 2nd Khalif, Umar (RA) ladies who came to the mosques were dressing very inappropriately, attracting the attention of other men and there was a good chance of affairs erupting. He consulted Ayesha (RA, Prophet's wife) and banned ladies from coming to the mosque. This is the reason, the imam said, that ladies should not be allowed in any mosque.

How true is this story? How much of it is an exaggeration? God only knows. Is this applicable today? In the 21st century, in the West (or even East). Is this real Islam?

At the end of his speech and the ceremony, I caught the imam and said that at the time of the Prophet (PBUH), ladies were allowed in the mosque. It is well documented that the Prophet used to shorten the prayers when ladies were there, in the mosque, with young children. What happened at the time of Umar is recorded in history. However, history is not all facts. It depends on who writes it, what are his own views about a particular issue, how far is he happy to exaggerate or suppress an event, how far is he happy to lie etc. I have read widely different accounts of the history of India's independence and the creation of

Pakistan. The historical events in Karbala (Iraq) have more than one version. Even the history of World War 1 and 2 is not all 100% facts.

The best example of how history can be widely different is that of Ibrahim (AS). The Muslim history says that Ibrahim took his son Ismail to be sacrificed, whereas Jewish history says it was the other son Isaac (A.S.).

You cannot and should not take decisions in today's world based on some historical event that cannot be guaranteed to be 100% true. Even if that event was true, the decision taken could have been for that time and place only, made by taking into consideration the circumstances at that time. It should not overrule common sense and general principles of humanity. Allah respects the whole of mankind, which includes women, as it says in Surah Bani-Israil, Surah No: 17, verse 70:

"We have honoured the children of Adam…and preferred them over many of our creation." The point to be noted is that women are included in the term "children of Adam". Just because they are different to men in their anatomy, physiology, endocrinology, psychology, etc., does not mean they should be treated as "low caste" and therefore not allowed in the mosque.

Women have been given great respect in Islam. Examples are Mary (R.A.), the mother of Jesus (R.A.), Pharos's wife, Khadija, Ayesha, Fatima (R.A.).

In his last sermon, the Prophet (PBUH) mentioned a great deal about women, how to treat them, respect them, men's rights towards them and their rights towards men.

I told this Imam that all the mosques in the Arab world allow women. The best example is the two holy mosques, one in Mecca and the other in Madinah. The Imam's answer was that Arabs do not know Islam; We (Asian maulvis) know the right Islam. I have heard this argument before, that Arabs do not know Islam; only Asian maulvis from religious schools from the sub-continent of Indo-Pakistan know the right Islam.

I asked the imam did he mean that the entire Muslim Arab world was wrong.

He did not answer Yes or No. Instead, he said, "Look, Doctor Sahib, you are a doctor of medicine. Whatever you say in medical matters, we will believe you without questions. We (Asian maulvis) are doctors of Islam, whatever we say about religious matters, you must believe without questions." He called himself Doctor of Islam, although he did not have a Ph. D in Islamic studies. He only had a certificate from a religious school in India. These religious schools (even in the UK) run within the mosques are totally unregulated. There is no government body keeping an eye on them, there are no Inspectors of schools. Each school promotes its own version of Islam (like this one which says that women are not allowed in the mosques).

However, these schools are still doing a good job in the sense that at least children are learning how to read the Quran and the essentials of prayers etc.

I have heard this argument many times from the maulvi that as medicine is for doctors only, engineering is for engineers only etc., so is religion for them. They say that whatever a doctor says in relation to a medical matter, we accept, same way whatever "We" say about any religious matter, Muslims should accept. "We" are the doctors of "Islam," he said, "In fact, you all obey me in prayers. When I ask you to bow down, you do; when I ask you to go in Sajdah (prostration), you do. So why not obey me when I say that ladies are not allowed in the mosques?" This argument was, in fact, his "ego's defence mechanism." He felt great calling himself Doctor of Islam. This showed his inferiority complex.

The imam said that medicine is for doctors only, engineering is for engineers only, law is for lawyers only, so is Islam for us (maulvis) only. This is totally false because:

I have many books on medicine and many books on religion. My brother is an engineer, he has many books on engineering and many books on Islam. My brother-in-law is a lawyer, and he has many books on law and on Islam. Does any maulvi have books on medicine and engineering and law? No–of course not. The reason is medicine is for doctors only, engineering is for engineers only, law is for lawyers only, BUT Islam is for everyone.

I have been hearing speeches from maulvis and imams in various mosques for many years. I can easily find so many flaws in their speeches and so many good points. I can comment both positively and negatively, I can give cross-references and say what other scholars have said on a given topic and how this differs from what a maulvi is saying. However,

If I give a speech to maulvis on the aetiology, pathology, pathogenesis, differential diagnosis, clinical features, and treatment of "Aspiration syndrome" or COPD (Chronic Obstructive Pulmonary Disease), or any other medical condition, can any maulvi comment on that? Can he give cross-references?

A lawyer or an engineer can deliver a Friday prayer sermon and lead the prayer. Can an Imam argue a case in a court of law? Can he construct a bridge? They cannot because it is not their field.

The reason I can comment on maulvis speeches and they cannot comment on my 'speeches on medical topics' is that medicine is for doctors only, but Islam and religious knowledge is for everyone. Anybody, who can read and write and has an interest, can gain religious knowledge. There are so many examples where people did not go to "madrasas (religious schools)" and yet gained enough knowledge in religion to be well known, e.g. Allamah Iqbal (the poet of the East), professor Meer Waliuddin of Osmania University, Hyderabad, India, Abdullah Yousf Ali, Ahmed Deead, Dr Zaker Nayek, Dr Israr Ahmed, both medical doctors, Dr Hameedullah (Paris), Gary Miller, now Abdul Ahad of Canada, Dr Maurice Bucaille (writer of " The origin of man and The Quran, Bible and science), etc. What these people have done, nobody qualified from a madrasah can do.

Maulvis say that as you cannot become a doctor just by reading medical books, similarly you cannot become an "Aalim (scholar)" just by reading religious books. What they forget is that medicine is a science and a skill. To take out an appendix needs knowledge and skill that is why you cannot become a doctor just by reading books. Whereas giving a speech in a masjid is simply a matter of knowledge, where is the skill here? Of course, Public speaking is an art, but it is never taught in madrasahs.

Feedback.

During my studies for my fellowship examinations (F.R.C.A.) in London, I had many well-known professors giving lectures on various topics. At the end of their lectures, they always give 'feedback' forms which ask about the quality, contents, presentations etc. about their lectures and a final question is "how can we improve our overall teaching?" Compare this with the speeches given in the mosques. People are not allowed to ask questions. I have been actively stopped to ask questions. Questioning a scholar (speaker) is regarded as an insult to him. It is a blind belief that a scholar is always right, so simply believe in whatever he says. They have no concept of 'feedback' to improve themselves.

Even if two speakers give totally contradictory views on a particular topic, we are still not allowed to ask questions. In my local mosque, two speakers were invited to speak on "Shab-e-barat" (Night of freedom). The first speaker gave half an hour talk on the authenticity and existence of Shab-e-barat. The second speaker gave a ten-second speech and said, "there is no such thing as Shab-e-barat." Nobody in the audience asked any question about this contradiction. I was not allowed either.

I can speak on many Islamic topics giving references from the Quran and other books. Can any maulvi speak on topics from medicine, law, and engineering etc.? Of course, he cannot.

Islam and its understanding are for everyone. *It is not a monopoly for maulvis.* Anyone can gain sufficient knowledge by reading books, gaining preliminary knowledge from teachers, asking people with the knowledge about matters he does not understand, referring to various books to understand a topic, doing research work, and thinking, reasoning and logic and knowing his limits. With self-motivation and dedication, he can understand Islam much better than those qualified from traditional religious madrasahs. He will not simply believe in everything given to him in the name of Islam. He will use common sense, and most importantly, will not say silly things in the name of Islam.

Conclusion: Islam is not a monopoly of Maulvis only.

Chapter Three
Muslim Scholar from South

Africa...Cure for Many Ailments

One day I was coming out of my local mosque, a member of the mosque committee stopped me and said, "Doctor Sahib (Sir)", a renowned scholar is coming from South Africa to give a series of talks in Ramadan. He is very good, very knowledgeable, he speaks in "English, you must attend his talks, he speaks in English."

This "Renowned Scholar" from South Africa is invited to give a series of talks every Ramadan. He speaks in English. For the majority of Asian mosque attendees, anyone who speaks in English is a highly literate, knowledgeable and renowned scholar, regardless of what he says. He cannot be wrong. He is an ocean of knowledge. To me, this is a pure "slave's mind". I am not the only one who thinks that it is a pure slave's mind' *Mufti Mohammed Taqi Usmani* of Pakistan, in his Urdu book, "Dunya mere Aagey...the world in front of me" on page 25, writes on this issue as well.

Every language is rich and beautiful, and you can express your thoughts effectively in any language. We should not be prejudiced against any language, like Hindi and Sanskrit are for Hindus' only, Arabic, Persian and Urdu are for Muslims only etc. I have passed three examinations in Hindi and I read and write Hindi without any problems. I have an A level in Arabic as well. Currently, I am studying an advanced Arabic course.

I have listened to this "renowned scholar" quite a few times. Most of the time, his talks are good and sensible. But whatever good and sensible things he (or any other Muslim scholar) says are already there in the holy Quran, one and only intact, pure, and perfect message from Allah. If you know your Quran well, and you have a thinking mind, ready to do some research, you do not need these "renowned scholars."

However, like most of these scholars, not everything he says is right. Below is an example:

In a Friday sermon, he talked about the benefits of *Wadhu* (Ablution, i.e., washing of hands, arms, face, cleaning head and washing feet before Muslim prayer).

He said that by doing Wadhu, you do not suffer from, in fact cure, high blood pressure and depression. He went into details of how by rubbing the sides of the fingers during wadhu, you stimulate the nerves in the fingers and the stimulus goes to the brain and cures high blood pressure and depression. Also, when you wash your head and the area behind the ears, the Mastoid process is stimulated to cure hypertension and depression. All this had no scientific basis at all.

Then he went on to say that some pharmacists and psychiatrists are "prescribing wadhu" to their patients to cure the two diseases. He said that "they" have done experiments to prove its validity. He did not say who "they" are? in which country "they" have done the experiments? In which scientific journal the method and the results of the experiments were published? in which country the pharmacists and psychiatrists are prescribing Wadhu for high blood pressure and depression?

This "renowned scholar" has no scientific background, does not know the criteria for the validity of any scientific experiment and its data and yet he is claiming these benefits of Wadhu. I have heard this sort of claim from other so-called "scholars" as well. Such claims do not exist and the Quran and Islam themselves do not make such claims.

After the Friday prayer, I wanted to ask this person only one question and that is, "In this mosque, many people regularly come to offer their prayers, they do Wadhu regularly, five times a day, they have been doing this for years and yet quite a few of them suffer from high blood pressure and some from depression. Why?" I know that they have hypertension and depression because they consult me from time to time about their medications and the side effects.

I could not go anywhere near this 'renowned scholar' as he was 'surrounded' by his devotees. Ultimately, I managed to get near him and said that I wanted to ask him a question. He said that he did not have time and went away. These people shy away from any questioning. They know that they cannot give credible answers to questions.

This scholar did not have time to answer my questions; he was rushing to other mosques to deliver the same sermon. He was touring the UK to give people his 'valuable knowledge'. God only knows how many people would stop their medications after listing to this scholar thinking that Wadhu alone would cure their illnesses.

In a separate incident, an imam of a mosque, whom I knew very well, stopped taking all his medications for diabetes and hypertension because some other religious scholar, more 'knowledgeable' than him, told him that he did not have diabetes or high blood pressure, all his symptoms were because he was possessed by an evil spirit, and someone had done a bad spell on him. He was advised by this 'knowledgeable' scholar to stop all his medications and chant some special words X number of times a day.

When this Imam told me about this, I strongly advised him not to stop his medications. He could chant the special words as many times as he liked, but "please do not stop your medications." The Imam did not listen to me, stopped all his medications, had massive bleeding in his brain and died, leaving a young widow and young children.

I sincerely hope that after listening to the 'benefits' of Wadhu by this South African scholar, people will not stop their medications.

We need to get rid of this culture of **'BLIND BELIEF'** in our Maulana, Maulvis and Scholars just because they have a particular outfit and appearance, carry 'a' certificate from 'a' religious school. They do say a lot of good things, but not everything they say is right.

Know your Quran well, and you will not have a blind belief in everything you hear and read.

Not just Muslims.

This culture of blind belief in the religious people is not unique to Muslims only. Below are two examples:

1. There was a Christian patient in my hospital suffering from cervical cancer who stopped her treatment halfway through, saying that there was a priest in Nigeria who, sitting there, was going to cure her through his spiritual powers.

2. There was another lady in my hospital in London, who was neither Muslim nor Christian, who needed surgery to deliver her baby. She phoned her spiritual leader in her home country to find out what was the auspicious time for the surgery. The spiritual leader gave her a time and she requested to have her

surgery at that time. We respected her wish, but it was very inconvenient for the doctors and the team and risky for her and her baby.

Muslims need to know the Quran well and understand it well. This is the only way to get rid of such 'ignorance' of blind belief in our religious so-called leaders and scholars.

There have been many incidences of blind belief in the religious leaders in every community, every religion. As I said many times, "It is very easy to fool people in the name of religion…Muslims are no exceptions."

Chapter Four
Muslim Scholar from India

I read a variety of books from a variety of authors. I listen to a variety of speeches from a variety of speakers. I have been doing this for many years. Now I am retired, I can write my own views about what I have been reading and listening to.

Whenever I sit down to read a book, I keep a red, a blue and a green pen with me. Anything I disagree with, I mark with a red pen, green marking is something very good and blue is for an average thing which is still worth reading. My reference book is The Quran. Anything which goes against the Quran is marked with a red pen. Green marking is for something good expressed in the author's way, but the origin comes from the Quran.

There was a renowned scholar in India who has written many books on various Islamic topics (a total of 800, includes books and booklets).

One of his books, "The life of Muslims", is very good. It is worth reading. I read this in the Urdu language; I liked it so much that I got a copy in English for my wife and children (they are born and brought up in London and they do not know Urdu). When I read this book, I felt very happy that the author knew the Quran very well and grasped the fundamental message of the Quran and has a thinking mind. Everything he has written in this book originates from the Quran. The author expressed and explained various topics in his own way, but the origin is from the Quran.

However, I read another book from the same author written in Urdu. The nearest translation of the name of the book in English would be "Deeds of the Quran". Everything written in this book, I marked with red. It is not worth reading at all. Anyone with a sensible mind reading this book would say that the author does not understand the Quran at all. He does not think.

Let us take just one example. One of the chapters in the book is:

"How to capture your local Jinn (sprit)."

The concept of spirit is in many religions, in different forms. It is a non-materialistic entity. In Islam, it is not the soul.

In this, he writes a procedure to capture the local Jinn. It includes verses from the Quran and some kind of exorcism. In my view, these verses are totally irrelevant. What he has not written is whether he himself tried this procedure? If so, was it successful? What did he do with the Jinn? Where did he keep the Jinn? What did he feed the Jinn with? etc. By the way, Jins (sprits) are invisible to human eyes.

During my training as a doctor in India and in London, I took part in scientific research, helped my consultants in clinical trials, established epidural service in Medway hospital, Gillingham, Kent, England, etc. As a person of science, I can say:

Criteria for the validity of an experiment/procedure:

There is a strict criterion for the validity of any experiment or a particular procedure. For example,

If I tell you that I have combined two metals in a particular way which resulted in a third metal which is gold, then for this experiment to have any validity,

a) It should be repeatable, i.e., each time I do the procedure, I should get the same result.
b) Anyone else doing the procedure in the same way, must get the same results.
c) There should be independent observers to verify the results.

This Indian scholar did not do any of this. He simply wrote the procedure of capturing the local Jinn. I am not writing the procedure here; in case somebody tries and develops psychiatric illnesses.

Another question that came to my mind is that why did he write this? Where did he get the information from? Nowhere in the Quran or Hadis (Prophet's sayings) has it said to capture your local Jinn. Why write something which is totally useless, has no value, and was never done by the Prophet (PBUH).

People who have '**BLIND BELIEF**' in our scholars will believe in this author because he is very well-known in the Indian subcontinent, even though he did not capture any jinn. The other danger is that such people (the blind believers) would believe in anyone who says that he had captured Jins, who could sort out all the problems of the people at 'a cost.'

Such things are common in the villages of India, Pakistan, and other Muslim countries. Probably, this happens in other non-Muslim countries as well. A few years back, a headless torso of an African boy was found in the river Thames and police ultimately traced this to exorcism in an African country.

In another incident, many years back, a Muslim woman, Ms A, in Glasgow, was jailed for life for killing another woman, M/s. B., who apparently was possessed by the Jinn. The woman who was jailed, Ms A, was regarded as a "very religious and knowledgeable" woman in her circles who knew "a lot". She tried to expel the Jinn, who apparently had possessed the woman, Ms B. In doing so, Ms A kept hitting Ms B so much that Ms B died.

I knew and have read many true incidences in the Indian subcontinent, where people (Muslims and non-Muslims), blindly following their religious Gurus, have done extremely horrible things, including having sex with a recently deceased woman in her grave to cure infertility and killing a six-week-old baby, born on a *Tuesday,* drinking some special drink in his skull–again for infertility. Why Tuesday? Because the Guru said so.

It is very easy to fool people in the name of religion. Muslims are no exception.

During my working life in the operation theatres, we have successfully investigated and treated (I.V.F.) many patients for infertility. So, if one is having problems of conception, I strongly advise her to seek medical treatment rather than go for such so-called religious people who claim to have special powers and can sort out all your problems at a hefty cost. The cost is not just money, but most of the time, it involves women sleeping with them.

If the medical treatment fails (sometimes it does), then it is better to be content with God's will than go to such people. If you just follow the general principles of, whatever your religion is, this should be enough as, 'being content with what you have'. This is an important general principle of all religions.

Coming back to this book, "Deeds of Quran", another chapter is how to treat a patient who cannot pass urine. The author has used a verse from the Quran, chapter 36, and verse No 34. In this verse, Allah is describing how He has created everything on the earth for mankind. One of the things is the flowing rivers and water springs. The author says that if you chant this verse and blow on the bladder of the patient, the patient will start passing urine (urine will flow).

The above two are only examples. This book is full of such things.

The 'scholars' of Islam can say and write whatever they feel like. There is no quality control.

The most important thing is that "you are responsible for your actions."

Authors and speakers on Islamic topics:

After the encounters with the two renowned scholars and reading and listening to various other 'scholars' (some of their sermons and writings are included in this book), I divide these scholars into two groups.

In **group A** are the scholars who say very nice and sensible things. You may not agree with everything they say, but they do not say anything which can be labelled as 'silly'. This group includes people like *Allama Iqbal, the poet of East, Professor Mir Waliuddin from Hyderabad, India, Dr Hamidullah from Paris.* Also included in this group are *Ahmed Deedat, Dr Zaker Naik, Abdullah Yusuf Ali, Adil Slahi, etc.*

In **group B** are included all those who say nice and sensible things, and yet something very 'silly' as well, as mentioned in chapters like, *Jins did It, chapter 14, page 99; MRI and tiger, chapter 6, page 69; Professor of physics and 666, chapter 5, page 66.*

I kept thinking about what the difference is between groups A and B?

My conclusion is that all the people in group A did not go to any religious schools; they had their normal, standard education. Whereas, all those in group B did go to the religious schools *only.* They did not take the standard pathway of education where they would learn subjects like maths, physics, chemistry and other sciences, sociology, history, geography etc. These subjects help in developing common sense, thinking, reasoning, logic etc.

For a long time, I stuck to this conclusion that it is the education in religious schools which take away the ability to differentiate between what is right and what is 'silly.'

However, I had to change my view when I came across two GPs, a consultant physician, an architect, an engineer, an airline worker, and a lawyer.

They all took the usual, standard pathway of education, and yet they said some very silly things in the name of Islam. For example, this lawyer, in his speech on a Pakistan Day function, said: "After the Prophet (PUBH), if anyone's example is to be followed, it is Jinnah's example." He completely ignored the companions (Sahaba, R.A.). Did he not read in the Quran what Allah says about the companions in Surah Al-Fatah, chapter No 48, last paragraph?

Does he not know this Hadis where the Prophet said that my companions are like stars, i.e., a shining example of Islam.

So, I was back to thinking as to what is the difference between groups A and B? My current conclusion is that in group A, people do not have a **blind belief** in whatever they read and hear. They **THINK**. They follow various verses of the Quran in which Allah asks mankind to think, ponder.

In one of the scientific journals, it is mentioned that the majority of people in the world do not use their full mental capacity. This includes memory, mental maths, common sense, thinking, reasoning logic, willpower, decision power, ability to draw a conclusion, learn from self and others experiences of life etc. These are the mental faculties Allah has given to man. Allah has created plenty of signs in the universe for mankind to think about and recognise Him as a creator. As it says in Surah Ale-Imran chapter 3, verse 190, 191:

Indeed, in the creation of the heavens and the earth, and in the alteration of day and night, there are signs for men of intelligence and understanding (they recognise the existence of Allah by these signs). They remember Allah at all times, contemplate about these creations and say, Oh our Lord; you have not created these without reason. Glory to you, save us from the hellfire.

A similar message has been repeated in the Quran many times.

There are two words used in these verses which need further discussion. One is men of understanding *and intelligence* and the other word is those who *contemplate (think)*.

These two faculties of intelligence and thinking have been given to everyone. It is a matter of using them. You do not have to have an IQ of 200+ or a champion of Mensa to use them. On the day of judgement, no one will be able to tell Allah that he did not find anything on earth through which he could recognise Allah. The fact is: He (Man) did not think.

Chapter Five
Professor of Physics and 6666

I was preparing for my fellowship examination (F.F.A.R.C.S.), and for this, I was attending a course at the Royal College of Surgeons, Lincolns Inn, London WC2A 3PE.

There was a fair amount of physics I needed to know for my examination and, of course, for my work in the hospitals.

A professor of physics came from Cambridge University to give a lecture on a particular topic. The class was full, around seventy students, who were all qualified doctors.

During his lecture, the professor wrote a particular formula on the blackboard. It was a long and complicated formula. Since I had prepared this topic beforehand, I noticed one mistake in the formula. I stood up and said to the professor, "Sir, there is a slight mistake in the formula." He asked me what the mistake was, and I told him. He said very politely that he would look at it at the end of the lecture, which he did and told me in the full class that I was right.

The professor **did not** tell me off, saying, "How dare you challenge me. Do you know who I am? I am **The** professor of physics from **The** Cambridge University. Do you know, or do I know?" No one from the class of seventy doctors came to take the side of the professor or told me off for pointing out Professor's mistake. The professor thanked me for correcting the mistake (a genuine human error).

Now compare the above with the following:

The Same-day in the evening, on my way home, I stopped at my local mosque to offer the evening prayer. After finishing the prayer in the congregation, as I was coming out of the mosque, I noticed a poster near the exit door. The title of the poster was **"Miracles of The Holy Quran"**. There were quite a few points, some clearly exaggerated. One of the points was that the number of verses in the Quran was 6666 and it is a miracle. This is clearly wrong.

One of the imams was standing near me. I drew his attention and said that it is totally wrong to say that the Quran had 6666 verses. The Imam got extremely angry with me and said, "How dare you say that it is wrong. Do you know who wrote this poster? Scholars from Jamia Noor-ul Huda, South Africa (a renowned madrassah in South Africa), how can they be wrong?

"Do you know more than them?" He was all huffed and puffed, angry face, red, popping eyes. Some other imams came to help him. They agreed with him that the scholars from such a renowned institute could not be wrong. The scene was becoming very ugly, so I walked out because The Quran says: Surah Al Furqan, surah no. 25, verse 63: *When ignorant people argue with you, say to them "Goodbye".*

The point here is not how many verses are there in The Quran. There are different ways of counting the number of verses in The Quran. Going by the commonest way, the total number of verses is 7339. Counting by other ways, it is different but well above 6666.

The main points here were:

1. **Manners**: The Imam got incredibly angry with me. He had a perfect Muslim outfit and appearance but no Muslim manners. Did he not know that in the Quran, Allah says: "Speak to people politely, softly, with manners.", chapter 2, verse 83, and chapter 17, verse 83 and chapter 41, verse 34 and many more. There are also many verses about controlling your anger, e.g., chapter 3, verse 134. There are many Ahadees (Prophetic sayings) on this topic as well.

The Quran also mentions the manners of dealing with a different opinion, the way to take criticism. Some verses I have mentioned above. In practice, Muslims are ready to argue and fight each other because they have different opinions. Once, a senior member of the preaching party (Tableeghi Jamat) told me that he would pray for me so that Allah could guide me to the right path. He looked down upon me. In his view, I was away from Islam. This is because I disagreed with him on an Islamic issue.

Compare the manners of imams with the manners of the professor of physics. He was a Christian, displaying very good Christian manners. There are so many common values between Islam and Christianity. Politeness and good manners are part of every religion and a matter of common sense. The professor realised that he was a human being and, therefore, likely to make mistakes. He and the students in the class were educated, well-mannered people. They were all highly educated and knew how to behave.

2. **Blind belief:** This is the usual problem with many Muslims. They have an absolute blind belief that whatever the speaker is saying is right. They are psychologically impressed by the speaker because he has "an appearance, a typical outfit" and a certificate from a religious school and speaks in English. He has quite a few titles before and after his name; somebody is "The ocean of knowledge", another person is "The wise man of the Muslim nation" or "The shining sun of knowledge" etc. He cannot be wrong. All these titles are given to them by their blind believers, not by any organisation/body who goes through their work and decides to give the title or not. Islamic literature has no 'quality control.'

3. **Homework.** Muslims themselves are not prepared to do any homework, i.e., study The Quran, and understand it and think, so that they can differentiate between right and wrong. One of the names of The Quran mentioned in The Quran is *Furqan,* which means criteria to differentiate between right and wrong. It is 'The' book that differentiates between right and wrong. Chapter 25 of the Quran is named "Furqan". The first verse of this surah says, "Glory to One (God) who sent down the Furqan, i.e., criteria on his servant, i.e., the Prophet, peace be upon him."

4. **Spread of the knowledge.** In Surah 17, verse 36 and in Surah 49, verse 6, Allah says that if you do not have the knowledge "for sure" about anything, then do not spread it.

Note: Surah 17, verse 36: "And say/pursue not that, of which you have no knowledge. Surely, the hearing, the sight, the heart, all will be questioned on the day of judgement."

"You believers; if a liar/evil person comes to you with a news, verify it, lest you harm others and then regret your actions."

Chapter Six
MRI and Tiger

I had made an arrangement with the management of the hospital, London E11, that I would take every Friday afternoon off as my half-day, so that I could do the Friday prayer in the mosque.

On a Friday morning, as usual, I was in the hospital before 7:30 a.m. The operation list was full. However, I cancelled a major case as the patient was not fit for the surgery.

I finished my work around 10:30 a.m. (instead of 1 p.m.). As I was coming out of operation theatres, I saw a notice that there was a lecture on MRI (Magnetic Resonance Imaging). The MRI scanner was recently installed in the hospital and the lecture was about how it works and the science behind it. It did not have a direct bearing with my work as an anaesthetist, but as I am very passionate about science, technology and 'general knowledge', I attend these sorts of lectures whenever possible. Knowledge is power, I believe in this. The pen is mightier than the sword, I believe in this as well. So, I attended the lecture on the MRI.

The lecture was very good. It explained the physics behind it. The use of an MRI, how it differs from the CT scan, its indications, and limitations etc.

As I was driving back home, I was praising Allah for how many things He has made and how He gave 'Man' the knowledge to make things work for him, how His signs are everywhere around us. It reminded me of a verse from Chapter 41, Verse 53, which says: *We will show you our signs in and around you…*

I realised that all these discoveries are made by the western world. Everything we use today is discovered and made in the western world. We call them infidels, unbelievers etc., but when it comes to science, technology, medical treatment, social security, benefits, and free treatment, free education etc., we look to the west. This country (UK) is fair and just to all its citizens without any discrimination. Allah has established kindness and justice in their hearts.

My thoughts went back to all the scientific discoveries over the centuries. Muslims did do scientific experiments and discovered quite a few things, but that was in the past. In today's world, Muslims are far behind in this field and other fields like industries, agriculture etc. When it comes to industrial advancement, we always hear about, the USA, the Western world, India, China, Brazil, but not a single Muslim country.

Coming back to the science behind the MRI, I was glorifying Allah for everything He has made and subdued them for mankind and gave man knowledge to use them. As it says in the Quran in chapter 31, verse 20:

"WE have subdued everything in the earth and the sky to you."

Meaning, use them for your benefit, for the benefit of mankind.

With all these thoughts, I came to the mosque (London E11) for the Friday prayer. The Imam stood at the pulpit and started his sermon:

"There was a *Murshid* (religious teacher). He knew some very special religious words. If you put a tiger's picture in front of this teacher, he reads these special words and blows on the tiger's picture, the tiger comes to life and comes out of the picture. When he reads the antidote words and blows on the tiger, the tiger goes back into the picture." (*It was becoming quite difficult for me to hold my laughter.*)

This teacher (the Murshid) had a student/disciple (Mureed). The teacher had taught the student these special words as well.

Now, both the teacher and the student set out to meet the king of the land. When they reached the king's courtyard, the king was busy talking to other people. He did not pay any attention to the teacher or his student. The teacher was very patient, but the student lost his patience. There was a picture of a tiger on the wall. The student read the special words in his mind, blew at the tiger's picture and the tiger came out of the picture, onto the floor of the courtyard. The tiger was wandering around in the courtyard everywhere, but nobody paid any attention, never bothered to know where did this tiger come from? The teacher got angry with the student that why he (the student) lost his patience. He looked at the student angrily. The student realised that his teacher did not like what he did. So, the student chanted the antidote words and the tiger went back into the picture. The king and other people in the courtyard still did not pay any attention to the teacher or to his student. The student again lost his patience. He again looked at the tiger's picture, the tiger came down and the whole process was repeated, again and again. Ultimately, the teacher and the student came back without meeting the king.

What rubbish this whole sermon was? In the morning, in the hospital, I listened to a genuinely nice lecture on how the MRI scanner works. In the afternoon, I listened to this wonderful 'enlightening' sermon.

After the prayer, I asked this Imam about where he got this story from and what was the lesson to learn from it?

He said that he read this story somewhere. Where? The answer was, "Can't remember".

(So, he read, so he believed).

I asked him as to what the lesson was, to be learnt? The answer was he wanted to teach the worshipers to have patience. I told him that the Quran has many verses about the virtues of having patience, with many examples like Prophet Job having extremes of patience during his illness. I asked him why he did not use these examples. The imam kept quiet, hoping for me to go away.

Saying this, this Imam has given some good sermons. I have seen this problem with many of these imams that they believe in everything they read or hear from others. They do not think if it is true, what is the authenticity? Does this make any sense? Whenever I asked them about the references of these stories, the answer is always, "I read somewhere, but I can't remember". They cannot differentiate what is right, what is wrong and what is silly.

Scholars or storytellers? Entertaining the crowd is an art and our religious scholars are very good at doing so. They come out with lots and lots of stories like these which are totally unauthentic, unbelievable, and sometimes have a fair amount of sex in them. So-called 'Islamic literature' and YouTube are full of such stories with the so-called 'scholars' of Islam.

Saying all this, there are some very good, sensible, real scholars who deliver very good sermons. They do not talk any nonsense. Examples are Nouman Ali Khan from the USA, Peer Zulfiqar Ahmed, Garry Miller, Late Ahmed Deedad, Adil Silahi, Yousuf Islahi, etc. These people are educated, they think, and they know their limits. The Quran describes such people as "solid in their knowledge (*Rasiqul-ilm), people with intelligence (Ulil-albaab)*"

Chapter Seven
"God is Very Kind to Mankind"

This verse appears in the Quran in many places, like chapter 16, verse 7, chapter 22, verse 65, chapter 2, verses 143 and 251 and many more.

I was watching a programme on TV about how much scientific research and advancement the west made between the Gulf war one and the Gulf war two. For example, according to this programme, in the first Gulf war, the fighter planes had the capacity to pick up an individual building to bomb. In the second Gulf war, they were able to pick up not the individual building but the window or the door of an individual building. The laser-guided technology was replaced by magnetic tunnel technology. The programme also showed the firepower the western world has.

I thought about this verse (God is very kind to mankind) and thought that the firepower which the western world has today, if the Muslims had the same power, given the status of the Muslim world, there would be a lot more atrocities in the world, many more killings of innocent people, much more destruction. Anyone who disagrees with their 'version' of Islam or any opinion which is against their opinion would be killed. According to a video I received on WhatsApp, more Muslims have been killed by Muslims than non-Muslims. Examples given in this video were Afghanistan and Syria.

Therefore, Allah is very kind to mankind by not giving Muslims the firepower which the western world has. The Quran teaches us how to accept a different opinion. If you think that you are right and the other person is wrong, The Quran tells you how to express your opinion. If the person/s disagrees, leave them to Allah. As it says in chapter 39, verses 3 and 46 *"Allah will make a final decision, on the day of judgement, in the matters in which we, disagreed with each other."*

One of the Maulanas (religious person) from the local mosque used to come to my house to teach my children some basic Arabic.

One day, when I came back from the hospital, this Arabic teacher had finished the lesson with my children and was about to leave. I greeted him, asked him how he was? Etc. He was looking unusually happy. I asked him and he said he was going to Mecca and Medina for Umrah (pilgrim). I said that was very good and asked him if he was going alone or with his wife. He gave me a strange look and said, "Doctor Sahib, what are you talking about? If you take women with you, it is all problems. Woman is nothing but problem. You should go alone so that you can do your prayers and supplications etc., very well. You take women with you; she will create nothing but problems. Women have only two places: the tip of your shoes and the kitchen. She has only two jobs, cook and produce children. "I got so angry with him that I asked him not to come to my house again."

God is really kind to me that I do not believe in such Maulanas.

My thought went to another Maulana in our local mosque. Once, he told me that he wanted to take a bulldozer and demolish all those Muslim houses which have televisions in them. In his view, watching TV was Haram (forbidden). There are many like him, making many things haram. Another Maulana in the mosque told me that if you do not wear a cap while offering your prayers, the prayers would not be accepted. Some mosques in Hyderabad, India, have appointed boys whose duty is to put caps on every worshiper's head who is not wearing a cap.

These people bring their own personal opinions in the name of *Shariya law*. If such people get power, they will bomb all the Muslim houses which have TVs, where men wear western clothes, where the women go to universities and go to work. This is their way of spreading what they call 'true Islam'.

God is really kind to us that such Maulanas are not in power.

It was a routine for this person (one who said that watching TV is haram) to stand at the exit of the mosque at the end of each prayer and tell everyone who was going out that watching TV is haram.

I heard him for few days and then one day I asked him: "Why do you think watching TV is forbidden?"

He said, "Oh, it has all dirty material. The way to eradicate evil is to cut its roots."

I said, "if this is so, all cars should be banned. People use cars to come to the mosques, people also use cars to commit sins as well. Since they use cars for the wrong purpose, cars should be banned, i.e., cut out the roots of the evil. Similarly, ban all kitchen knives. One can use a knife to cut vegetables, but the same knife can be used to kill someone. Therefore, ban all the knives, eradicate the evil from its roots."

Then I asked him some questions of general knowledge, what was happening in the country, in the world etc. His knowledge was close to zero. I told him that by the grace of Allah, my general knowledge is very good, 90% of this general knowledge comes from TV. I watch the news, documentaries and all the educational and scientific programmes like Panorama, Sky by night, Click and many more. If you have a strong concept of 'Accountability', you will not watch any dirty programmes. Who is your real enemy? Christians? NO, Jews? NO, Hindus? NO. Anyone else? NO. Your real enemy is inside you, who persuades you to do wrong, to watch wrong, control this enemy, rather than bomb/bulldoze Muslims' houses.

This person in the mosque who said that watching TV is haram reminded me of another religious person I came across when I was unmarried. He had a typical Muslim appearance. He got me a marriage proposal. The girl was completely uneducated, so I declined her. When this person asked me the reason to decline her, I told him that I wanted to marry an educated girl. He was shocked to hear this. He said, "Doctor Sahib, what are you talking about? girls should not be educated. Your wife should be a house bond wife. Keep her at the tip of your shoe". When I heard this, I controlled my anger and told him not to come to my house again. There are still some people who have these kinds of views. These people have no idea about how important worldly education is, especially science and technology. They are uneducated, want to remain uneducated, and want to keep other Muslims uneducated. They think this is all Islamic. They think that education, especially western education is bad. Yet when they fall ill, they go to the hospitals which run, based on western education and research. They fly in the planes for Hajj and for visiting sacred places. These planes came into existence because of western knowledge and research. They use mobile phones to talk to their relatives in their home countries but do not think for a single second, "Who made this phone? Who developed the technology? Views expressed by such people are totally un-Islamic."

When the Prophet (PBUH) said, "Seek knowledge, even if it is in China." He did not say that it is for men only. He also did not say that here knowledge means religious knowledge only. Allah, in many places in the Quran, mentions "people of knowledge", "people of wisdom". He does not say that here people mean men only.

Educate your children, boys and girls. Give them the best of both worlds by giving them fundamental Islamic knowledge as well as good worldly education.

Remember this prayer in the Quran for your spouses and children: "Oh our Lord, make our spouses and our children the coolness and comfort of our eyes and grant us grace to lead the righteous (make us an example for others)." Chapter 25, verse 74.

For children to be the coolness and comfort of the eyes of their parents, they must be good in both the religion and in the world.

They are not the coolness and comfort of your eyes if they are good Muslims, offering their five daily prayers, fasting throughout Ramadan, etc. but they are uneducated, unskilled, unemployed, unemployable, and unable to stand on their feet. Similarly, they are not the coolness and comfort of your eyes if they are highly educated, have good jobs but millions of miles away from the religion, involved in everything which Islam forbids.

You have to strike a good balance between these two things. There are verses in the Quran which ask you to gain knowledge of the religion as well as the world and use this knowledge for the betterment of yourself and for the world.

One of the many reasons I left the preaching party (Tableeghi Jamat) is their slogan: "Work for the world as much as you have to live here, work for the hereafter as much as you have to live there."

The interpretation I was given for the first part of the slogan was that since you live in this world for few days, you do not have to do much. This straightaway implies, "No education, no need to find a job, no need to make your life decent and comfortable. After all, one day you have to die".

I have been listening to the Friday sermons, Ramadan special talks, and many other talks from our religious leaders for the last sixty years. Not even once any speaker highlighted the importance of worldly education. Yet when I read the Quran, I found that many verses imply for us to gain worldly knowledge, especially knowledge of science and technology. For example, chapter 62, verse 10 it says, *"...spread out over the land and look/search for the bounty of Allah."* Agriculture, growing crops, minerals, knowledge to construct buildings etc., are all bounty of Allah, but to use them, you need knowledge. That is why there is a B.Sc., M.Sc., PhD in science. Minerals are the bounty of Allah. How to extract them from the earth, how to purify and how to make things from them, all need knowledge of science and technology. In chapter 57, verse 25, Allah talks about Iron, its strength and says that there are benefits in it for mankind. However, to get its benefits, one needs knowledge. Knowledge of how to extract it from the earth, how to purify it, how to makes things from it and most importantly, how to convert it into steel.

The verses in chapter 3, last verse, chapter 8, verse 60, and chapter 4, verse 71 cannot be put into practice unless we have a very high quality of knowledge in science and technology.

I wonder why all the so-called scholars of Islam I have been hearing in the last sixty years did not think of it?

Chapter Eight

And the Patient Said:
"You Don't Know Who I Am."

All religions teach us to be humble, down to earth. All religions teach us to spend some of our money on those who are less fortunate.

"Do not walk on the earth with pride/arrogance. Allah does not like those who are proud of themselves". The noble Quran, chapter 31, verses 18 and 19. The fourth Khalif Ali (RA) said, "We all come from earth, so we all should be down to earth."

I was a junior doctor in Scotland. One day I was in my clinic. From the place I was sitting, the river Clyde was clearly visible. It is a big and deep river.

One patient walked in wearing a kurta and salwar (baggy Asian clothes). I took his history, did measurements of his blood pressure, pulse, blood sugar, and did an ECG. He was suffering from high blood pressure and diabetes. He was quite an overweight person and from his history, it was quite clear that he did have no concept of exercise and dieting. Since it was a new case, I consulted my consultant and prescribed him the necessary medications.

The patient looked very worried. I told him that he had neglected himself quite a bit, but not to worry, take these medications and do some exercise. I advised him about dieting as well. He still looked quite worried and asked me if he could go private. In those days (1980s), private hospitals were not very common. I told him that it was not necessary for him to go private. The private sector gives the same treatment as the NHS hospitals. In fact, the NHS hospitals are far better in providing specialist treatment. They have lot more facilities than private hospitals.

I also told him that the private treatment was very expensive. When he heard this, he got very angry and said: "Dr Sahib, you don't know who I am. Do you know how much wealth I have? You see this river Clyde? If I throw my money in this river, the river will stop flowing."

He regarded that the "expensive private treatment" was an insult to him. I calmed him down and asked him to go home and take the medications I had prescribed. I gave him another appointment after three weeks.

Three weeks later, the patient did not turn up. We sent him another appointment. He still did not attend the hospital.

Further investigations by the social services department revealed that this patient went back to his home country (Indian subcontinent), went to visit some relatives in a village, had a heart attack and died due to lack of medical facilities.

"There was no profit to him from all his wealth and all his gains" Chapter 111, verse 2.

All the wealth he had hoarded, with which he could stop the river Clyde to flow, was not of any help to him. The Quranic concept of wealth is that you earn, use for necessities, and spend on others who are less fortunate than you. "*Those who hoard the wealth, gold and silver and do not spend in the path of Allah, give them the news of a severe punishment in the hereafter.*" Chapter 9, Verse 34. Similarly, in chapter 104, Verses No 2 and 3, it says, "*One who hoards the wealth and keeps counting it, thinking that this wealth would make him last forever…*"

We all make mistakes; we all are sinners. However, as the Prophet (PUBH) said, "the best sinner is one who repents."

Chapter Nine

It is OK to Cheat Whites...Really?

1. One day, I was coming out of a mosque in London E11. After the mid-day prayers, one of the worshipers, who knew me very well, took me to a corner in the mosque, took out some papers, and asked me to sign some declaration. I asked him what that was about. He said that it was to make an illegal immigrant, legal. I told him that he had just finished his prayers, this is a mosque, a sacred place and you are asking me to sign some papers which are totally false. His answer was, "Oh, doctor sahib (Sir), to help our Muslim brothers, it is OK to cheat whites."

As this was a mosque, I had to control my anger and frustration on his fraudulent behaviour. We had a long conversation. Briefly, it was like this:

His view was that since these 'whites' have ruled over the Indian subcontinent and sucked out all the wealth from India, it is OK to cheat them. You are helping your Muslim brothers anyway.

I told him that there are quite a few points we need to discuss.

Firstly, I asked him: "Do you read Quran?" His answer was, "Yes, every day." "Do you understand what you read?" I asked him. "NO", the answer was, loud and clear.

This is the problem with the majority of Asians. They read The Quran but do not know what they read. I told this person that this means you do not know all those verses in the Quran where Allah asks you to say what is right, what is just and fair. For example, in chapter 33, verse 70, 71, Allah says:

"Oh, you believers, be aware of Allah, say what is right. Allah will make your deeds whole and sound and forgive your sins. He, who obeys Allah and His Messenger, has already attained the great victory."

I told him that there are so many verses like this in which Allah asks you to be fair and just with everyone, regardless of his/her beliefs, even if the verdict goes against yourself, against your parents and family. Allah is always reminding us about accountability on the day of judgement.

This person said, "Oh, no, but these people (whites) have ruled over India for so many years." I told him that this, no way, gives him the right to cheat them. If these people ruled over India, it is the fault of our forefathers to let them rule. Muslims ruled over India for centuries, much longer than the Britishers; does this mean that Hindus should cheat the Muslims in India?

This person said, "But they, the Britishers, also killed lots of people, including Muslims in the incidence of Jallianwala Bagh, how do you explain that?" I told him to read Indian history. Delhi was 'ruined' seven times, every time by Muslims. The mass killing of King Naadir Shah is well known, in which thousands of innocent people lost their lives, how do you explain that?

Then I told him that if he had read The Quran, knowing what he was reading, he would not have asked me to sign these false documents. I told him that this country (Britain) had given us so much, we should always be well-wishers and loyal to this country and its people. Think of all the free health care in the NHS, free education in schools, free meals, the various benefits etc. I know the value of the NHS because I worked in the NHS for more than forty years. In this country, all your rights are given to you without any hustle. I remember, when my father retired in India, it took him more than a year to sort out his pension because he refused to bribe the officials who were dealing with his pension. However, when I retired in the UK, I had no problems getting my pension.

We need to be loyal to the country where we live. This is Islam.

We have no right to cheat anyone. This is Islam.

You say what is right and just. This is Islam.

You do not favour 'your people' because they are 'your people'. This is Islam.

You do not forget ACCOUNTABILITY. This is Islam.

If you are overwhelmed by the feeling that your forefathers were treated badly by the forefathers of 'these' people (British) or you feel that some of the 'these' people are treating you badly, then remember this verse from the Quran, chapter 41, verse 34 and 35, *Repel evil with good, then the one who hates you will become your good friend.*

2. Do not take his side:

One morning, in London, when I was coming home from the mosque after the morning prayer, I witnessed a car accident.

Car A was being driven by an old English gentleman and behind his car was car B, driven by an Asian man. A cat was crossing the road, so car A suddenly braked. Car B was too close to car A, and it could not stop in time and crashed into car A. It was clearly the fault of the driver of car B. Both the drivers came out of the car. The old English gentleman was looking very worried and confused. I approached him and said that I had witnessed the accident and I would be a witness for him if necessary. Seeing this, the driver from car B started talking to me in Urdu (Indian language) and said, "Do not take his side. He is a white man. You should be on my side; I am your Muslim brother." and he started saying the same thing as the one in the mosque.

I wanted to tell him everything which I had said to the man in the mosque. When I refused to take his (car B) side, he (the driver) looked very unhappy with me; he declared me a Kaffir (unbeliever) for taking the side of a white man.

However, not all Muslims are like the above two. Those who understand The Quran do not behave like the above two.

When my sister retired in India, she got some lump sum and she wanted to buy a flat with that money. She found a flat. The seller was a Muslim. A price was agreed between the two parties, but at this stage, nothing was in writing. Some other people approached the seller and offered him a much higher price than what was agreed with my sister. The seller refused to accept the higher price saying that his words were valued more than the extra profit he was offered. He was following various verses from Quran with regards to keeping up your promises, like chapter 5, verse 1, chapter 23, verse 8 and many more.

He was the true follower of Islam. There are many examples like this.

To be fair, there are good people in every religion because the general principles of all religions teach humanity. A) An English lady gynaecologist, a true Christian, took my side in a disciplinary committee hearing because she knew I was right.

B). Hindu, Muslim riots are common in India. However, there have been incidences where good people from each community saved each other's lives.

C) In my early days in the UK, Dr Nayak, a Hindu, went out of his way to help me.

D) According to a Pakistani Christian, Imran Khan's cancer hospital treats whoever walks in. Religion, caste, creed etc., is not asked.

Chapter Ten
How, Why, When, Where, What

I have been listening to various sermons and speeches from various imams and other religious speakers for more than sixty years. I feel that most (not all) of our Imams are good in what they have learnt in the religious schools in the Indian subcontinent, but they cannot relate their knowledge to the present day's issues affecting the Muslim communities. For example, in the Friday sermons, or Ramadan speeches, they talk about stories that happened centuries ago. These are the stories that I have been listening to since my childhood. God only knows how many of these stories are accurate. The only 100% true stories are those given in the heavenly books. Our imams and speakers never talk about current affairs, what is happening in the world and around them etc.

When I talk to these people, I always stress the importance of science and technology and other education pertaining to this world. I always say that the salvation of Muslims here and the hereafter is Islam and science. What Muslims practice in the name of Islam is just performing routine rituals and they are right at the back of the queue when it comes to science. How many Muslim countries have a space programme? None. How many are counted as 'industrialised nations'? None. With the nation's wealth, Muslims make skyscrapers and compete with each other in doing so, but they make all these with borrowed technology. The day their wealth is finished, they will have begging bowls in their hands.

On one such occasion, I was talking to an imam of the mosque (London E11). This imam, like most of the imams from the Indian subcontinent, had only religious school education. He had never read mainstream subjects like maths, physics, chemistry etc.

I was explaining to him how science has evolved.

The basis of science is 'the' philosophy; the questions of How, Why, When, Where and What. I gave him some examples, like:

When Sir Isaac Newton was sitting under an apple tree and saw the apple falling on the ground, he asked himself, "**why** this apple fell down on the ground? Why didn't the apple go up?" He kept thinking about this, and his research ultimately led to the discovery of gravity, gravitational forces and finally "Newton's laws of forces". Today's jets and rockets fly because of this discovery of the gravitational forces, laws of forces and how to overcome the gravitational force.

I gave him another example of how the radar was invented. Well before the Doppler Effect was discovered, the scientists observed the bats. They asked themselves, "**How** do the bats find their way when they have very poor/non-existing vision?" The research led to the discovery of the reflected sound, now called the Doppler Effect. This is the basis of the radar system.

I gave him other examples like the discovery of penicillin, the discovery of the X-ray etc. These were again based on why, when, where, how etc. The imam kept nodding his head. He did not ask any questions. It became quite clear to me that he was unable to understand what I was saying.

Friday Sermon

The next day was Friday. This imam came on the pulpit and started his sermon by saying, "In Islam, there is NO such thing as Why, When, Where, How, What. You should simply believe whatever we tell you to believe." Then he went on to say that your "Iman" (faith) is in danger if you start asking questions. He was referring to the belief in the unseen. I felt very angry and frustrated. If he had told me beforehand what he said in his sermon, then I would have explained to him that:

This philosophy of How, Why, When, Where and What is essential to the scientific experiments, research, inventions and development. It applies only to those things which themselves or their effects can be felt by five human senses. For example, you can do experiments on light (electromagnetic radiation) because it can be sensed by the human eye. This is the faculty of sight. An X-Ray is also a light (electromagnetic radiation), which cannot be sensed by the human eye, but its effects can be sensed. Magnetism cannot be seen or felt by human senses, but its effect can be. Similarly, we can hear the normal sound but not the ultrasound. But the effects of the ultrasound can be felt by human senses.

We cannot see infrared light, but its effects can be sensed.

Allah has given humans the faculties of sight, hearing, smell, taste and touch, with limitations. For example, we can see the normal light but not every light, like ultraviolet or infrared light. But we can sense the effects of those unseen lights.

"And He taught Adam the names, i.e., knowledge, of all things..." 2nd chapter, verse 31.

Although Allah has given us these senses with limitations, He also gave us the knowledge to extend these limitations. For example, our sight can see up to a limited distance. With the help (scientific invention) of the telescope, we can extend this limitation.

Similarly, we can hear sounds from a certain distance. With the invention of telephones and mobile phones, we have the facility to hear sound from anywhere on the planet.

Although with the help of the scientific knowledge which Allah gave us, we can extend our limitations to our physical faculties (e.g., telescope), these extended physical faculties also have limitations. For example, even with the strongest possible telescope, we cannot see what is behind a wall. With the strongest possible hearing aid, we cannot hear every sound, like ultrasound or sound, from any distance.

Therefore, our extended faculties also have limitations.

Faculties of thinking, reasoning, logic, common sense.

As sight, hearing, etc., are our physical faculties, similarly thinking, reasoning, logic etc., are our mental faculties. As our physical faculties have limitations, similarly, our mental faculties have limitations as well.

As with our knowledge, we can extend our physical faculties, similarly, with the knowledge, we can extend our mental faculties as well. As the extended physical faculties have limitations, similarly, our extended mental faculties also have limitations.

Belief in the unseen. The 3rd verse of the 2nd chapter of the Quran mentions the belief in the unseen. This belief in the unseen is well beyond our extended mental faculties. The philosophy of How, Why, When, Where and What has limitations and does not apply to the belief in the unseen. This is the reason why all heavenly books, including The Quran, were sent down by 'Inspiration'. They are not the results of human thinking, reasoning, logic etc.

In fact, in the Quran, there are so many verses in which Allah says: "Indeed, in these are the signs for those who think, who ponder, who have the knowledge, people with wisdom".

Therefore, Allah expects us to use all these faculties because He has given all humans these faculties. He also expects us to know our limitations.

When I told this imam about "Why, When, How, Where and What," I definitely did not mean to use these to question the existence of God and other unseen things like Angels.

Our imams are very respectable people, they lead the prayers. Most of them are very humble, meek, down-to-earth and pious people. Other people ask them about their 'problems'. God has given them a very special position. They can address hundreds of people at least 54 times a year (52 Fridays + 2 Eids). However, if they are not aware of current affairs, do not have enough knowledge about the world in which they live, they cannot give practical advice which is within the Islamic framework. For example, once I asked a mufti if the pension contributions are "Zakatable (Obligatory charity)", He could not give me sound advice because he did not know about the state pension, company pension, private pension and how the system works.

In the 21st century, we have many problems which did not exist in the olden days. One, I mentioned above (pension contribution and Zakat). There are so many others, like, a Muslim pilot taking off from Bombay for New York at Fajar (dawn) time, completes his journey in fourteen hours. During this time, i.e., fourteen hours, he sees two sun rises. Is he going to do five prayers in fourteen hours while flying the plane?

Similarly, once a medical student told me that he was consistently missing the 2nd lesson after the lunch break because he had to go for afternoon prayer. One of the doctors was brought to the discipline committee because he was consistently not answering his bleep on Fridays between 1 pm and 2 pm.

In future, as science progresses, there will be more issues. For example, the ESA (European Space Agency) is developing an aeroplane that would fly from London to Tokyo in two and a half hours. If you (a Muslim) leave London at Fajar (dawn) time, you will reach Tokyo at their Esha (night) time. When would you do your three daytime prayers? Three donors' embryos is another issue that will make us ponder. Our religious leaders and true scholars (not the storytellers) will have to think a lot.

To give religious advice on such issues, one must have a very good, working general knowledge. This comes by regularly listening to the news, reading newspapers, watching documentaries etc.

When Tim Peak, the British astronaut, went to the ISS (International Space Station), I watched the whole process. In the evening, when I went to the mosque, I told one of the regular worshipers how exciting that was. The answer I got was, "it is nothing to do with us. It is nothing to do with Islam."

On another occasion, I brought up the topic of Brexit. Maulvi sahib told me that it was nothing to do with us. We have come in this world to keep chanting "Allah, Allah."

As I mentioned earlier, I have great respect for our imams. All I want from them is to gain the world's knowledge as well.

When they have this knowledge, only then they will realise the importance of **Why, When, Where, How, What.**

Chapter Eleven
Ram Gopal and Malik Husain
(not the real names)

"Man gets what he works for." Chapter 53. Verse 39.

Studies and exams are not easy. Whatever you are studying, you need to work hard, have a lot of patience and perseverance. To gain something, almost always, you need to lose something.

If doing a basic medical degree (MBBS/ MBChB) is like walking on a flat surface, then doing a post-graduate medical degree, i.e., fellowship (F.R.C.S.), is like climbing Mount Everest. I know this because I went through this procedure in London.

I was working in Scotland. I was the senior-most among the junior doctors. I had just passed the fellowship examination. My consultants were very happy with my work and with my overall performance.

There were two more doctors in the department, Ram Gopal (Hindu) and Malik Husain (Muslim). When they were appointed, they were told that they must study and pass the fellowship exams. It gives the department a good name. My consultants told me to look after them and help them in their studies. They both started studying for the fellowship exams. I told them that it was not easy; there was a lot of physics, chemistry, calculations, in addition to normal subjects. I told them that they had to be working very hard, be steadfast and be perseverant.

After about two months, Malik Husain told me that he was finding it difficult and was giving up his studies. I told him that this was not the right attitude: "If others can do it, you can do it". Malik Husain still did not want to continue with his studies. I told him that giving up and losing hope was very un-Islamic. Islam encourages its followers to be bold, courageous, never give up, do not lose heart and fight back whatever problems they have in life.

I told him the verse in chapter 12, verse No 87:

"…and never give up hope of Allah's soothing Mercy: truly no one despairs of Allah's soothing mercy, except those who have no faith". Here, Yaqoob (Jacob. A.S) is giving advice to his other sons when sending them to go and look for Yousuf (Joseph) and his brother (Benjamin).

I told Malik Husain about the advice Luqman (AS) gave to his son in chapter 31, Verse 17: "Face with patience (and courage, and consistency and perseverance) whatever problems you have in life. Indeed, doing so is among the great tasks." I told him that there are so many other verses in The Quran on this topic*.

However, Malik Husain did not listen to me and gave up his studies.

Ram Gopal continued with his studies and passed his exam.

(*Every religion asks its followers to be bold, patient and not to lose hope in God's mercy.)

One of the consultants in our department went on maternity leave. I was given her position as a locum consultant. My consultants asked me as to who was the deserving candidate to be given a senior position, Ram Gopal or Malik Husain? I told them that Ram Gopal deserved the senior post. He was hard-working, punctual, and sincere and he had passed the exams.

Now the situation was that I was the consultant, Ram Gopal was the registrar, and Malik Husain was the Senior House Officer (lower than the registrar).

What goes on in the operation theatres is a very complex, delicate and 'risky' process. All the members of the team must be highly trained, skilful and must have the appropriate knowledge of their roles. There are senior members and junior members. Juniors need to seek advice from seniors if they are not sure about any particular issue.

On some occasions, Malik Husain had to seek advice from Ram Gopal and had to do what Ram Gopal told him to do. Ram Gopal was a very humble and meek person, never showed off that he was a senior to Malik Husain, and he had passed the exam. However, Malik Husain did feel that he was taking 'orders' from Ram Gopal.

One day Malik Husain told me: "Look Dr Khan, I am a Muslim, I do my five daily prayers, every day I read The Quran, at least one chapter, I fast throughout Ramadan, yet Allah had bestowed His mercy on a Kafir, i.e., unbeliever (Ram

Gopal). I have to listen to and obey him. Is this fair?" I told him, "Yes, it is very fair." He got annoyed as I supported Ram Gopal and not him.

I asked him, "You read at least one chapter of The Quran every day, but do you understand what you read?" The answer was, as expected, "NO, I do not understand what I read". This is a very big problem with most Asians. They read Quran, but they do not know what they read.

I told Malik Husain that had he read the Quran, knowing what he was reading, he would not have given up his studies and he would not have said that it was unfair that Allah had bestowed His mercy on a Kafir. Allah has set up some rules to run this universe. They apply to everyone, regardless of his faith. One such rule is: "You work to achieve something, you get it, and you make a mistake, you pay the price." You (Malik Husain) did not work for exams, so you did not get it; you made the mistake of giving up hope, so you paid the price. One of the attributes of Allah is He is fair and just; chapter 3, verse 18. What happened to you and Ram Gopal is Allah's fair and just system.

Malik Husain was also upset that I recommended Ram Gopal for a senior position. I told him to read the Quran, this time with meaning, and read Chapter 33, verse 70, in which Allah says to the Muslims to say, "what is right, just and fair". Also, to read chapter 4, verse 135, which is:

"Oh, you believers! Stand out firmly for justice, even if it is against yourself, against your parents, against your kin, or against the rich or poor."

Reading without knowing the meanings: A big problem with Asians is that they can read The Quran without knowing its meaning. Even children who are doing Hifz (memorising the whole Quran) do so without knowing the meanings.

This reminded me of another incidence:

18690 rewards.

If you go to any Asian mosque between the middle (Asar) and after sunset (Maghrib) prayers, you will find many people reading Quran. Most of them do not know the meaning of what they are reading. Once I got an explanation for it: One day I was coming out of the mosque after Maghrib (after sunset) prayer, one of the worshipers who knew me very well, told me that between the Asar and Maghrib prayer he had earned 18690 (or a number in thousands) rewards. I was surprised. I asked him to explain how he counted his rewards. He said that he had read X number of verses from the Quran, then counted the number of letters in those verses and then multiplied them by 30. The result was 18690. Then he went on to explain a Hadis in which the Prophet (PUBH) told his companions that on each letter of the Quran you read, you get ten rewards. This is how he got 18690 rewards. I told him that while the Hadis is very true, the Prophet was speaking to the Arabs whose mother tongue was Arabic. They knew what they were reading. For us, we need to know the meanings as well (and learn Arabic language).

He smiled and said a phrase in Urdu, which means:

"Eat your mangoes, do not count the trees." This means as long as you get the rewards, don't bother about meanings.

Such people, who read Quran but do not know what they read, end up like Malik Husain, having unreasonable expectations from Allah.

Unfair and Unreasonable Expectations

Clearly, Malik Husain had unfair and unreasonable expectations from Allah.

Allah is not going to get someone through his exams just because he is doing his five daily prayers, fasting in Ramadhan, and reading Quran every day. Allah is not going to give someone a senior position if he does not deserve it.

I have come across some other incidences where people had unfair and unreasonable expectations from Allah:

"A Muslim man was accused of sexually assaulting young girls. The case was going on in court. I knew this person and his family very well. The family decided to do a ceremony of chanting *Isem-a-Azam* (Allah's greatest name) 150,000 times. They believed that by chanting Allah's name, they would win the case. I was invited to take part in this ceremony. I refused, saying that it would not work. It did not. The person was found guilty and was sent to prison.

It is a common practice among Asian Muslims that whenever they have any problem, they totally rely on solving the problem by chanting some words. This does not work. They must be reasonable for their expectation from Allah.

Chapter Twelve
Cracks in the Walls of the Mosque

Friday sermon in London: The Imam comes on the pulpit (Minbar) and starts:

"Once upon a time, there was a mosque whose walls had many cracks in them. There was a church opposite the mosque. The building of the church was very posh, good looking without any defects or cracks in it.

One day, the priest from the church came to the mosque and asked this imam why the mosque had so many cracks in it." The imam said, "in our Quran, there is a verse which says that if this Quran had been sent on a mountain, the mountain would have crumbled. Since this mosque had many copies of the Quran, that is why the building had so many cracks.

The priest laughed and walked away. The imam felt insulted, came out of the mosque, gave a dirty look at the church and the church building came down crumbling."

What nonsense.

After the sermon, I went to this imam and asked him that there are so many mosques in this world and so many houses which have copies of the Quran in them, why do they not have cracks in their buildings. The imam started looking here and there, hoping that I would go away. When I did not go away, he said that he read this in a "book". So, he read, so he believed.

Someone who was listening to our conversation later told me: "If you want to understand Islam, keep away from such maulvis".

This imam qualified from a very well-known madrassah in India.

The actual verse is in chapter 59, verse 21, which says:

"Had We sent down this Quran on a mountain, you would surely, have seen it humbling itself and cleave asunder for fear of Allah. Such are the parables which We put to mankind that they may think."

It was clear to me that this imam completely misunderstood the verse and believed whatever he read in a "book", not realising that the writer of the book was a storyteller and not a scholar.

The same imam, one day after Maghreb (after sunset) prayer, was sitting near the exit of the mosque, looking at the people going out of the mosque. The imam was looking very sad. I asked him why he was so sad. He said: "Look, Doctor Sahib, look at all these people who are leaving the mosque. I have so much knowledge, but no one wants to benefit from my knowledge."

Fortunately, such imams are rare.

Chapter Thirteen

Women Suffer in Every Community

1. We are civilized, we are advanced

This incident happened in the late 1950s in Hyderabad, India. What was not acceptable in Indian society (especially in Muslim culture) at that time is probably acceptable now in 2021. The reader will have to go back to 1950s India to realise the actions and reactions of the people.

I start with a verse from the Quran:

"...Allah knows and you do not". This concept has come in many places in the Quran. Allah is the one and only who has the final, pure and perfect knowledge and wisdom.

Religious principles, which include "Do and Don't do", have reasons which we may not understand fully. However, if we do not follow them, the consequences can be disastrous.

In the 1950s, when my father retired in Hyderabad, India, from the post of Director of Higher Secondary Education, he got a lump sum. He wanted to buy a house. In those days, there were no estate agents, no building societies, and no mortgages. The houses for sales were advertised in the newspapers. People usually paid the entire amount in one go, as they saved for this all their working lives.

My father found one house for sale. The owner of the house, Mr Hasan, a Muslim, asked for X amount as the price of the house. The lump-sum my father had, was slightly less than the asking price. Hasan had some other potential buyers who were happy to give the asking price, but they were running around to arrange loans. Hasan was in a hurry to sell the house, so he agreed to sell the house to my father, with less than the asking price.

My father got suspicious as to why Hasan was in a hurry to sell the house. In those days, there were no solicitors and no surveyors who would investigate if there were any problems with the houses, in relation with the councils, with its structures, foundations, ownership etc. The buyer had to investigate all this by himself. My father did these investigations as to why Hasan was in a hurry to sell the house. The story which came out was as follows:

Hasan, in the 1950s, was very well qualified and had a very good job which gave him an above-average income. He had a beautifully decorated house, all the luxuries of life and apparently a beautiful wife.

It was routine of Hasan that every Saturday night, he would invite his male friends to his house and play cards with them till late at night. When he used to play cards with his friends, his wife used to feel left out and lonely. As the custom was at that time, she used to stay inside the house, in a different room. Hasan felt guilty and asked his wife to come and join in with them (he and his male friends) and play cards. The wife flatly refused. Hasan kept insisting and ultimately, the wife gave in to the pressure and started playing cards with his male friends till late at night.

There were occasions when Hasan was shopping on Saturdays and came late to his house. He told his wife to invite his friends into the house in his absence and look after them.

This happened several times.

When Hasan's relatives and well-wishers heard about this, they told Hasan that what he was doing was very wrong and un-Islamic.

Hasan laughed at them and said: "We are civilized, we are advanced, and we are not backwords like you".

The Saturday routine was going on as usual. By this time, the wife was very free with Hasan's friends.

At the end of one working day, Hasan came home in the evening and did not find his wife. He thought that she probably had gone shopping or to visit a friend of hers. The night had come and gone, the next day had come and gone; the wife did not come home. Hasan tried to search for her but without success.

Ultimately, it emerged that she had run away with one of Hasan's friends and was in his house. She demanded a quick divorce and a quick settlement of her portion in the house. This was the reason that Hasan was in a hurry to sell the house.

Hasan, with his worldly gains, pride, and position in society, had forgotten some fundamental principles. He did what he should not have done, i.e., encourage his wife to mix freely with his male friends. This principle is not just unique to Islam. Other religions like Hinduism also have similar restrictions. It is called "Laxman Rekha".

In Asian culture in general and, especially in Muslim Asian culture, the wife almost always gives in to husband's (and in-laws) pressure.

The attraction between males and females is natural. There is guidance in religions about how to behave with the opposite sex.

In the Quran, it says in quite a few places that if someone is doing something wrong, Allah gives him a respite to correct himself. However, if he does not correct himself, and keeps doing wrong, then Allah appoints "Shayateen" on him who glamorise his actions and justify to that person that what he is doing is right. This is the reason Hassan said to his well-wishers, "We are civilised, we are advanced, we are not backward like you."

Question: How far a wife should resist if her husband asks her to do something which she does not want to do? Which she considers un-Islamic. Should she put her marriage at risk? What comes first, marriage or principle?

Can Hasan blame his parents for not giving him fundamental Islamic education?

Is Hasan ultimately responsible for the breakdown of his marriage?

What Hasan's wife did, was it natural? Would any other woman do the same?

Answer: The Islamic answer is clear. It is not permissible for the wife to obey her husband in anything which is clearly haram (Haram is a term used to define those things which are clearly not permissible, e.g., adultery).

The attraction between men and women is very natural. This is how Allah has made us. There have been cases where the biological sisters and brothers were separated at birth/ childhood. They grew up separately, and in their adulthood, when they met, they developed a sexual attraction for each other and had intimate relationships. I know at least one case where they got married.

Allah has set some rules, regulations to prevent such attractions leading to adultery/incest.

In the Quran, Allah clearly says whom you can /cannot marry, Surah 4, Verse 22-24. He also mentions the manners of entering into houses, especially in women's presence, chapter 24, Verses 27 onwards. Other than this, He also says:

"Do not go anywhere near adultery." Chapter 17, Verse 32. This means do not get into any such circumstances/situations where you are likely to fall into adultery. Clearly, Hasan put his wife in this situation, in the name of "we are civilized, we are advanced".

In the 21st century, the majority of working people cannot avoid working with members of the opposite sex. There is nothing wrong with this. However, Allah gives you some guidance, for example:

"Keep your gaze down.", chapter 24, Verses 30-31. This is to safeguard you from falling into a situation where you are likely to commit a 'haram' act.

These rules and regulations, which Allah has put to run a **'clean'** society, should not be taken as 'restrictive', but they are there to protect women. People who follow these rules should be proud of them, rather than feel that they are 'backwards'.

Similarly, free mixing of men and women on a social basis is prohibited in Islam. At work, you cannot avoid it. In my 45 years of life as a hospital doctor, I never had a situation where I did not have a female colleague working with me. As long as you keep yourself within the Islamic boundaries, you will be fine.

On the same note, shaking hands of men with women and vice versa is not allowed either. In chapter 48, Verses 10 and 18, the Prophet is taking an oath of loyalty from the believers. In the explanation, it is written that the Prophet used to take the hands of companions into his hand while taking the oath. However, in chapter 60, verse 12, the Prophet is taking the oath from women. In the explanation, it is written that he never held any woman's hand while taking the oath.

2. Human sacrifice

Two thousand years ago, it was a custom in Egypt that each year a beautiful, young, virgin girl was sacrificed in the river Nile, to keep the Nile god happy.

Why not a boy or a man?

There have been cases of human sacrifice in the Indian subcontinent. The victim was always a girl/ woman. The idea was to get God's blessings for a big project. Was the god not happy with a male sacrifice? Why did it have to be a woman?

3. Buried alive. Burnt alive. No rights. No inheritance. Used. Married to Quran.

Before Islam in Saudi Arabia, most female new-borns were buried alive. Those who were lucky to be alive were used as 'things'. They had no rights, not allowed to inherit anything left by fathers or husbands. In fact, they were 'items' to be inherited.

In the name of **'Sati'**, in India, widows were burnt alive along with the dead bodies of their husbands. In England, in the name of **'witches'**, women were burnt alive. **'Chained wives'** are those who are divorced legally, by the law of the land, but not given a religious divorce, so that they are in limbo. Neither they have husbands, nor can they remarry because they do not have a religious divorce.

Although the practice of Sati is abolished in India, the practice of **'prabhudasi'** still continues in some Indian villages. Although made illegal by the Indian Government, Prabhudasis, according to an Indian true crime programme, Crime patrol, episodes 610 and 611 and also by Google, are young girls who were devoted to God (married to god) but in practice were used as prostitutes. This was practiced many years ago, now illegal by the Indian government but in some rural south Indian villages, still practiced.

There have been cases where businessmen used their wives, against their wishes, to 'entertain' the clients to get the business (Crime Patrol dial 100, episode 104 and 105).

On the 5 March 2017, an 'Inside Out' programme was broadcasted on BBC, titled *'Outcaste wives'*, showing the plight of Indian women.

Some time ago, there was a programme on TV named *'Brides of the Quran'*, where young Asian Muslim girls were married to the Quran. They stay unmarried all their lives but still fulfil their physical needs illegally (the aim of marrying the Quran is to keep the family's wealth within the family, otherwise it will go away with the girls).

Not enough dowries.

Ever since I could read, in India (the 1950s) I remember reading, on and off, cases of brides being tortured/burnt alive for not bringing enough dowries when they got married. There have been such cases in other Indian subcontinent countries, including Muslim countries.

Although the Indian government has made it illegal to demand dowry, the practice still goes on. According to Crime Patrol from India (true crime stories), on the 9 April 2018, until two years ago, every hour, a girl was murdered in India, for not bringing enough dowries. Their only fault was that they were born female, in a poor family.

"For which crime, they were killed?" Surah (chapter) 81, verse 9.

Shreya courts.

The most complaints in any Shreya court in England is from women, either against their husbands for neglecting them or against their fathers and brothers for not giving them their rightful share of inheritance.

Three seconds' divorce: Although it is totally in contrast to the Quranic teachings, a Muslim man, allowed by Muslim muftis, can divorce his wife in three seconds just by saying *"Divorce, Divorce, Divorce"*. However, if the wife wants to leave him, it is a long battle in the court that takes months. Last year (2017) the Indian Supreme court has made it illegal for Muslim men to divorce in three seconds **(the practice of three divorces)**.

4. The broken arm

Once I had a patient (non-Muslim) in a London hospital who came with a badly broken arm. I asked her how old the fracture was. She said it was four weeks old. I asked her why she was coming now. She said, "I was in India when I broke my arm. My mother-in-law did not let me go to the hospital. My husband did not/could not say anything. I came to London last night, so I am here in the hospital today."

It is always the woman who suffers most.

5. Possession by an evil spirit

There have been many cases in the Indian subcontinent where the diagnosis for a mental illness or for 'acting' was/ still is, straight away diagnosed as "possessed by an evil spirit". The 'doctor' who diagnoses this possession is a 'well respected' religious person with no medical or any education. He does some exorcism and gets rid of the evil spirit. The family is very happy, and the 'doctor' is paid well with money and goods.

In all the cases, the person possessed is a female. Nobody ever thinks why an evil spirit does not possess a man.

Even in the Hollywood film "Exorcist" (1973), the main character, possessed by the evil spirit, is a girl.

There have been cases in the Indian subcontinent and one in Glasgow where during the act of exorcism, the girls were so badly beaten that they died.

Here again, it is women who suffer.

6. Forced marriages and honour killings

In almost all the cases of forced marriages and honour killings, victims are women.

7. Gender pay gap

This is a hot topic in early 2018 in the UK. The businesses and organisations were forced to reveal the pay difference between men and women employees. In the majority of cases, women were paid less than a man for doing the same job (businesses do have a point that women take more time off than men for pregnancy and delivery). I am not an economist, so I do not know the answer to this point raised by businesses. However, here again, it is women who suffer.

8. Domestic violence

Even in the 21st century, domestic violence prevails in every society, regardless of whether the society is in the developing world or developed world. During the Coronavirus pandemic, 2020/2021, domestic violence against women had increased.

The developed and developing world is seen in view of the materialistic achievements and not in terms of good and kind human behaviour. The vast majority of victims of domestic violence are women.

(When I was working in the ENT department in Bishop's Stratford, in Essex, in England, I had an 84-year-old man with an injury to his external ear. His mother-in-law got angry with him and threw a saucer on his face).

What creates good and kind behaviour in a person? The answer is good religious education. However, this cannot be the only answer because there are people I have come across who do not believe in God and yet they are very kind and considerate, very meek and honest. Is it genes? Or surrounding? Or upbringing? Or anything else?

A psychologist is the right person to answer this question. For me, a good religious education is the answer, whatever your religion is.

Question: How far children should go to obey their parents? Below are the two incidences.

9. Two husbands

Once, in a London hospital, I had a young Asian girl who came for the termination of pregnancy. While talking to her, she said she was going home next week, to get married. I was shocked. She smiled and said in Urdu/Hindi, "I know why you look shocked. I have a boyfriend here in London, my parents are not happy for me to marry him. They have chosen a boy from home. I have never met this boy in my life. Even my parents had not met him. Just in one phone call, my marriage was settled. I cannot convince my parents that I do not want to marry him, so I am going there to marry him, to keep my parents happy. When I come back to London, I will have two husbands, one at home and the other outside the home."

Any decent man, regardless of his religion, will not ask his wife/children to do something against their religion/culture and wishes. However, if he does, then the wife/children need to consult someone sensible in the family/friends. There is much help available in western countries. This approach poses a big risk to married women, especially in the Asian community, as their marriage could be at risk for not obeying their husbands/mothers-in-law.

10. Emotional blackmail

I know at least two cases in Hyderabad (Muslim families) where the fathers emotionally blackmailed their children to do what they wanted, regardless of their children's wishes. The father's standard sentence was: "Do as I say, otherwise I will divorce your mother".

Here again, the poor mothers (women) were the victims, in addition to the children.

Such people who treat their wives and children badly are frustrated and angry of their failures in life. Since wives and children are 'weak', especially in the Asian community, it is easy to take out the frustration and anger on them.

All religions teach to respect women. Allah in the Quran and the Prophet in his last sermon mentioned to respect, protect, and treat women nicely.

For any man, no matter how great he is, his paradise is under the feet of a woman, i.e., his mother.

11. Be modern

In the 1960s, in Hyderabad, India, 'A' Muslim doctor got married. The girl was well educated, apparently, very pretty with long hair (long hair are a sign of beauty in Indian culture). The doctor was very happy.

The doctor passed the necessary exams to go abroad and went to a western country. A few months later, his wife joined him. Living abroad, soon, the doctor forgot his roots and values.

Then the doctor realised how 'backward' his wife was. He started telling his wife to be 'modern'. The first thing to go was her long hair, cut to the neck length in a beauty parlour. However, the wife resisted initially but then gave in to the pressure.

In Indian culture, especially among Muslims, when the girl is given away in marriage, she is told to be obedient to her husband and in-laws and do as she is told to do.

The next thing to go was her Indian clothes. Her Saree and blouse were replaced by 'modern' clothes, short and tight. The wife obeyed this as well.

When she was told to come to parties and mix with other men freely, this was the limit for her.

She did not run away with another man but was divorced for being "too backward, not understanding the modern ways."

Here again, a woman suffered due to her husband's views.

12. Mother's sacrifice

What a mother can do for her children, no man can match it. The following are a few true stories:

a) A woman in her mid-twenties was pregnant. Three months into her pregnancy, she was feeling extremely unwell. Blood tests showed that she had Leukaemia (blood cancer).

Doctors told her that she could start treatment 'now' and survive, but the treatment (chemotherapy) would kill her baby.

The second choice was she could continue with the pregnancy, but then she would die within months of delivery.

She took the second choice and died three months after the birth of the baby. Only a woman can do this.

b) A woman was crossing the road with her baby in the push chair. From her left side, a lorry was coming quite fast. It was clear that the lorry was going to run over the push chair. The baby's death was eminent. The woman pushed the push chair quite hard to the other side of the road and, in doing so, was run over by the lorry. She died instantly. The baby survived.

It takes a mother's heart to do so.

c) In the 1950s and 60s India, bacterial infections were quite common, like typhoid, diphtheria, cholera, tetanus, etc., fatalities were common too. I lost my elder brother, 16 years old, to typhoid.

I had diphtheria three times. On the third time, it was very serious.

A new therapy was introduced recently. Horse serum with anti-diphtheria antibodies was to be injected into me. This had some serious side effects. In those days, there was no ECG, pulse oximetry, end-tidal CO2 monitoring, etc.

I was told to lie in bed still for twelve hours after the injection of the horse serum. My mum was told to watch me continuously for 12 hours.

The injection was to be given in the late evening. It was the month of September. Manson rain was causing havoc. As my mum was coming to the hospital from home, the bridge over the river between the house and the hospital developed big cracks. Police stopped everyone from using the bridge as it could collapse at any time. My mum was walking to the hospital. She told the policeman that she was happy to take the risk. She had to go to the hospital, as I was to have the injection. She crossed the bridge, came to the hospital, stayed next to me for twelve hours, from 9 pm till 9 am, without a break.

Only a mother can do this.

No wonder why God has put paradise under the feet of mothers.

d) Watching various animal documentaries, I noticed that even in the animal kingdom, the way mothers look after their babies, fathers do not.

Note 1. To be fair with men, although they do not do as much as the mothers do, they do bring sustenance to the house. Their efforts are largely unnoticed.

When a child is hungry, it is a mother who puts food in his mouth. When the child is dirty, it is a mother who washes her and puts new, clean clothes on him. The child remembers this. The child never thinks, where did she get the food from? Who bought it? Who got the new clothes? Where did the money come from?

That is why, when the children grow up, they have more bonds with mothers than fathers.

In a quarrel between a father and mother, the children almost always take the side of the mother. Here, the man is the victim.

Note 2. Traditionally, 'Man' is exposed to the 'chronic stress' of life throughout his working career. Whereas a 'Woman' is exposed to the 'acute stress' of life, i.e., periods, pregnancy, delivery, postpartum, nursing and looking after babies, school runs etc. at a time of her life when she is physically young, fit and healthy. By the time she is in her middle age, children are grown up and independent. Now, a woman can relax, whereas the man in his middle age is still carrying on with his job and associated stress.

This is the reason that stress-related illnesses like high blood pressure, diabetes, angina, M.I. (myocardial infarction, meaning heart attack), cancer etc., are more common among men. Women, with their hormonal makeup, are less likely to develop cardiovascular diseases at a young age. However, with more and more women coming into working life, the trend is changing.

13. Man 'who wanted son' pushes wife and two daughters into well in India, killing 8-year-old child

Shweta Sharma
Mon, 7 June 2021, 3:10 pm

The man pushed his wife and two daughters, including an infant into the well (AFP via Getty Images)

14. Sacrificed to win the lottery.

10-6-2021. Danyal Hussein, 19, killed his two sisters Bibba Henry and Nicola Smallman, because he made a pact with Demon, to win the lottery. He promised demon to sacrifice six more "women only", every six months if he wins the mega million super jackpot. The case continues in London.

Comment: Women suffer in every community. Why in every human sacrifice, it is always a woman? Similarly, why Jins always possess a girl/woman?

15. 12-06-2021. Another victim of honour killing.... Of course, a woman.

In northern Italy, a Pakistani family has disappeared. Police suspects that the family killed their daughter who refused a "forced marriage" to someone in Pakistan. Police thinks that the family has fled to Pakistan. The girl's cousin has been arrested in France and extradited to Italy.

Comment: Islam is totally against "Forced marriages" and gives full freedom to the girls to choose their life partner. It is the local custom and culture which people associate with Islam. I wish Muslim study Islam i.e. The Noble Quran.

16. 5th July 2021. Red button service, BBC (world). Dowery in India. World Bank Researchers went through 40,000 marriages in India, which took place between 1960 & 2008. In 95% of these marriages, dowery was paid although it is illegal since 1961. *My comments:* This social evil, which often leads to domestic violence and death (murder or suicide) does not end on the day of marriage, although the dowery had been paid. It lasts for the rest of the life of woman. Those Indians who left India and moved to the Western World still carries the same mentality. An Indian friend of mine (doctor working in Glasgow), once told me that whenever he is short of money, he asks his wife to get it from her father. She had to.

Chapter Fourteen
Jins (Evil Spirits) Did It

1. This was a speech from a well-known, Arabic speaking 'scholar'. This speaker is an engineer as well. This speech was given at a religious function in London. The topic was "Jins" (Sprit, non-material entity, created from fire).

Some of the things the speaker said were from the Quran, and of course, there is no dispute about it. Other things were totally unauthentic. Then he narrated one incidence, which is as follows:

The speaker went to his hometown in his country, Egypt. In the night, he was sleeping in a flat on the first floor. In the middle of the night, there was a big bang in the compound. All the residents woke up and went down. They found the compound wall collapsed. They call the police and fire brigade who called the people from all the utility companies, i.e., gas, electricity, telephone, water etc. These people found no reason for the wall to collapse. They declared that the collapse was not due to any gas leak, or electrical fault or water leakage etc. Everyone was puzzled. Our speaker, being a great 'Muslim scholar', declared that Jins did it.

Nobody questioned him as to how he knew that Jins did it. Why did they do this? As usual, they had blind belief in the scholar and were happy that finally the mystery had been solved.

As I have said many times in this book, it is easy to fool people in the name of religion, especially Muslims.

2. Something similar happened in India. No cause of the fire was found. The residents of the home called a religious person. He came, gave a panoramic look at the house, and declared that Jins caused the fire because the residents did something which angered the Jins. People were happy with this verdict. The religious person received his gift (fee), and it was a happy ever after ending for everyone.

Now compare the above incidences with the following incidences:

1. In Yorkshire, something similar happened, i.e., a compound wall collapsed. Gas, telephone, electricity, water, etc., companies sent their investigators, who found no reason for the wall to collapse. The council appointed a team to investigate further. Their investigations found that once upon a time, the land on which the wall was built was a dump. People used to dump their refuse in that dump. Once it was full, it was closed. Sometime later, the ground was flat, and the wall was built there.

With time, the rubbish in the dump started rotting, producing Methane gas. As more and more gas was being produced, the pressure in that 'closed container' was increasing. At one point, the pressure was so much that it ignited the gas and caused the wall to collapse.

2. Another incidence in England:

A woman's house caught fire. The fire started from the front door. The investigators found no fault with the gas, or electric short-circuiting or any other reason for the fire. They kept investigating and found that:

It was peak summer. The front door was made of glass, which had additional decorative pieces made of glass. These decorative glass pieces were quite thick (convex). Behind this glass door was a curtain made of thin, inflammable material.

At a particular time of the day, the sun was very sharp and was shining directly on the glass door. The decorative pieces served as 'convex lenses', focused (concentrated) the sunlight on the inflammable material of the curtain, burnt it and started the fire.

As a physics student in my school in India, I have done these kinds of experiments under controlled conditions. It is perfectly possible to burn paper, or a piece of cloth with the help of convex lenses, in the peak summer, when the sun is very sharp.

Conclusion: It is about time our so-called scholars of Islam stop blaming Jins for every unexplainable thing, stop misleading Muslims and start believing in science.

Chapter Fifteen
"OK...OK...But No Heart"

"They ask you about the Soul. Say, the soul is by the command of my Lord. You are not given knowledge about it but very little." Surah: 17, Verse: 85.

I have spent about forty-eight years of my life working in hospitals. Out of this, more than forty-three years were in the operation theatres and in the ICU (intensive care units), resuscitation rooms, labour wards and acute trauma.

One problem which is common in the ICU is the organ donations from Muslim patients. Muslims are very happy to receive organs but not happy to donate.

Some time ago, during my C.P.D. (continuous professional development) courses, I attended a course at the Queens Medical Centre, Nottingham, and one of the topics was "organs donation". The speaker was an English intensivist. He asked a question: "Is organ donation allowed in every religion?" All the class said: "Yes, it is allowed in every religion, except in Islam". I stood up and said that in my understanding, it was/is allowed in Islam as well. The speaker agreed with me and said that in the 1980s, there was a conference of Muslim scholars in Kuwait and in that, all the scholars agreed that organ donation was/is allowed in Islam.

In a London hospital, I had a young Muslim boy who had a car accident with a severe head injury and was brought to our ICU. We kept him on the breathing machine (ventilator). After few days, we realised that he was not going to survive. Apart from his brain, the rest of his body was perfect for organs donation.

We started negotiating with the family for organ donations. As usual, the family refused. As I was the only Muslim doctor in the ICU., it came to me to convince the family, especially the father, to agree to donate his son's organs. I had a conversation with the father on more than one occasion. The summary of those conversations are as follows:

I asked the father why he was refusing to donate his son's organs. He said, "Oh, Doctor Sahib, it is forbidden in Islam". I asked him how he knew that it was forbidden in Islam. He could not give a clear answer and said that he heard that it was forbidden. I told him that it was not forbidden and gave him the reference to the conference of Muslim scholars in Kuwait. He was still reluctant. Then he came out with another point in favour of his refusal. He said that if he agreed and the organs were taken from his son's body, then on the day of judgement, his son would rise from the dead without eyes, without lungs, and without other organs. He would not be able to see, walk, talk, drink water, etc.

I told him that nothing like this would happen, as Allah has power over everything. He would bring the body intact. Then I told him about Prophet Ibrahim's (A.S.) conversation with Allah, Surah: 2, Verse: 60. In this, Ibrahim asks Allah as to how He brings the dead back to life. Then Allah asks him to take four birds, cut them into pieces, put the pieces on different mountains and then call them. Ibrahim did that and the birds came with intact bodies. This is Allah's power.

The father seemed to be convinced. He consulted his family and said: "OK...OK, but no heart". I asked him, "why not the heart?". He said that because the soul lives in the heart, therefore, "No Heart". I gave him a verse from Surah: 17, Verse: 85, in which Allah says, "They ask you about the soul. Say that the soul is by the command of your Lord, and you are not given knowledge about the soul, except very little". The father seemed more convinced.

I gave him another verse from Quran, Surah: 5, Verse 32 in which Allah says: "Whoever saves a human life, it is as if he has saved the entire humanity and whoever destroys a human life, without a valid reason, it is as if he has destroyed the entire human race".

Then I went on to explain to him more. I said, "You live in a house, which is very well decorated. It has got everything in it. A time comes when you are leaving the house forever. You are never ever going to come back to this house. Then what is wrong if other people use some or all the good, intact things which you have left in your house? It is a help to them. Allah will give you a reward for helping others." He agreed with me and finally and happily, without any pressure, agreed to the organ donation.

I asked him a final question, "If your son were alive and needed an organ/s transplant, would you take it from others?" "His answer was, without any hesitation, "yes, of course".

This is a problem with many Muslims. They are happy to take but not happy to give. I have come across some Muslim families who agreed to organ donations but put the conditions that the organs should go only to Muslim patients. This is illegal and unethical. They come out with reasons like, "if we give our eyes to a non-Muslim, he may see things with our eyes, which are forbidden in Islam." Or the recipient may drink alcohol with the help of "my organs".

When asked, "if you needed an organ/s would you take from Muslim patients only?" The answer was clearly no. In a desperate situation, they are happy to accept organs from anyone, regardless of his beliefs and habits.

A very different approach

However, I had another case of organs donations from a Muslim patient, with a *very different approach.*

A young boy was involved in an accident with a head injury. In the ICU, he was on the ventilator. A few days later, it was decided to turn off the ventilator, as it was quite clear that the boy was not going to survive. He was a perfect candidate for organ donation.

We asked the family and they agreed (very rare for a Muslim family to agree straight away).

I was the consultant on call that night. I went to the ICU, and before taking the boy to the theatre to remove his organs, we called the father and mother to come and see their son. It was around 1 a.m. I watched the father and mother. The mother almost fainted, but the father's behaviour was amazing. He was standing on the right side of the bed. His eyes were crying, and his tongue was praising Allah and reciting Quran. In between, he was consoling his wife, the mother of the boy. His left hand was holding his wife, who, otherwise, would have fallen to the ground. His right hand was holding the hand of his son, the 'brain dead boy'. It was a very touching scene, at 1 a.m. in the ICU. The only verse that came to my mind at that time was the last part of the 2nd Surah, which says, "Oh our Lord, do not put us through the tests which you have put others before us. Oh, our Lord, do not give us the burden which we cannot bear."

I am an educated and professional person. But that night, I had a practical, spiritual lesson in the ICU. from a non-professional, little educated, black collar/no collar, Bangladeshi worker. This lesson was a practical demonstration of patience, trust, gratefulness to Allah, remembrance of Allah and standing by his wife in the most difficult times. We can learn from anyone, older, younger, educated, uneducated, man, women, poor, rich etc.

I gave the parents enough time to spend with their 'clinically brain dead but biologically alive' son. Next time when they would see him for his funeral, he would be biologically dead as well.

Finally, I took the boy to the theatres around 2 a.m. By 6 a.m., all his organs were removed.

By the next day, his organs were functioning in different human beings in different parts of the country, giving the recipients new life.

"Whosoever saves one human life it is as if he has saved the whole of mankind …" Surah 5, verse 32.

This boy (and his parents for agreeing to donate their son's organs) saved nine lives (Two eyes, one heart, two lungs, one liver, one pancreas and two kidneys).

As human beings, we can help each other, regardless of our faiths. No religion is a hindrance in helping others, irrespective of faith. This is the reason one of the recipients of Zakat money (obligatory charity) could be non-Muslims (Surah 9, verse 60).

The Prophet (PBUH) said: "Best among you is one, from whom other humans are benefited." He did not differentiate between Muslims and non-Muslims.

Chapter Sixteen
Medical Issues Discussed in the Mosque

I know only two doctors who are medically qualified, and they serve as the imams of the mosques as well. They are doing a great job serving the community in more than one way. They do not discuss any medical matters in their sermons.

However, there are some imams who are not medically qualified. They have not seen any mainstream school in their life. The only schools they have been to are the religious schools. Yet, in the mosques, they discuss medical matters and advise the attendees. Almost all their advice has no medical grounds.

1. In the chapter "Scholar from South Africa", I have discussed his advice in detail.
2. Organ transplant In the chapter "OK. OK, but no heart" I have discussed another problem in detail.

I know one 'religious person' who was on the heart transplant waiting list. When the heart became available, he refused to accept it, saying that organ transplants are haram in Islam. Now his quality of life is very poor. This is the only case I know where the person refused to take the organ. Most Muslims are happy to take but not to give.

Not all imams and Muftis (jurists) agree that donating/receiving organs is permissible in Islam. Their followers have a blind belief in them and follow their advice, i.e., do not donate (but in a desperate situation, take).

3.   Post-Mortem.

One day, I was about to come out of the mosque; after the mid-day prayer, the imam announced: "In Islam, post-mortem is haram. There is a petition about this, near the exit, please sign this petition on your way out." He did not say where he got this information from? Has he himself done any research on it? Has he seen any post-mortems? Does he know the indications and contraindications of a post-mortem? Does he know the benefits of a post-mortem?

I stood near the exit to see who was going to sign. There was a long queue. Everyone was eager to sign. None of them asked the Imam about the source from which he got this information. They all had, as usual, blind belief in the Imam.

Later, I asked this Imam about the source of his information. He said he got it from "The Muslim Council of Britain, (MCB)." The imam himself put no thoughts of his own. He simply believed whatever the MCB told him.

I have heard this argument before that, in Islam, a post-mortem is forbidden. They relate it to the old tradition of 'body mutilation' in the days of ignorance, before Islam, in Arabia. The victorious army used to cut the body parts (ears, nose etc.) of the dead soldiers of the opposite army. The Prophet (PBUH), being mercy to mankind, forbid this practice. He asked his people to bury the soldiers of the opposite army with respect and dignity, without any body mutilation.

Today's post-mortems do not involve body mutilations. I have attended post-mortems. It is done with respect to the dead person and the body is returned to the family, intact and with full respect. By doing a post-mortem, doctors find the cause of death, any foul play and learn more of the disease which killed the person. This knowledge they use for scientific research to improve the treatment of the disease. This way, the dead person contributes to scientific research, which leads to the service of humanity.

X-ray post-mortem: Sometimes, instead of doing a standard post-mortem, it is possible to take an X-ray of the dead body.

Not all deaths go through a post-mortem. It is better to leave it to the doctors to decide if the deceased needs a post-mortem and, if so, which type.

I wrote a letter to the MCB asking for their reasons for declaring post-mortem, haram. I did not get any reply.

4. The difference between Unani and English medicine

In one of his speeches, the imam (London E11) discussed the above topic. He said that there are two types of medical treatments, Unani (Greek) and English. He completely ignored the "Ayurveda (ancient Indian)" and "Homoeopathic medicine". The imam went on to say the differences in the two types of medical treatments, how the diseases are caused by either "Cold", or "Warmth" and the treatment of diseases caused by "Cold" is through "Warm" medicines and diseases caused by "Warmth" is through "Cold" medicines. He did not give any example of any disease caused by cold or warmth nor any example of medicines used.

Much of it was totally unauthentic. Then the imam went on to discuss the *poisonous matter* in the body causing diseases and said that every disease is caused by the poisonous matter. He did not know that his poisonous matter is "sepsis". He did not know that not all diseases are caused by sepsis. He was going on and on about the treatment. I found it unbearable and walked out of the mosque.

The danger here is that the blind believers in such imams would go for treatments prescribed by such imams and pay the price. The following is an example.

5. Treatment of high blood pressure

One day when I was coming out of the mosque, I met a regular worshiper. I knew that he had medical problems, so I asked him how he was. He said that he was suffering from high blood pressure. I asked him what medications he was taking. He said, "nothing, I am treating my blood pressure with water." I was very surprised. Then he went on to explain that if you keep drinking water, you get rid of the "poisonous matter" which is causing high blood pressure. Once all the poisonous matter has passed through the urine, the blood pressure is cured. Obviously, this is not true.

If you have any medical problems, please consult your doctor, and follow his advice.

6. Antibiotics in honey

On 9 September 2018, I watched a YouTube programme presented by Mufti Tariq Masood of Pakistan.

He was discussing the good and bad effects of conventional antibiotics and antibiotics in honey. How the standard antibiotics kill the bad and good germs and honey antibiotic kills only the bad germs. As far as I know, he is not a doctor. Therefore, whatever he said, he probably got from google or read some so-called 'Islamic literature' and did not understand it very well.

There is no scientific proof of what he said. However, honey does have wound healing properties, but the mechanism of action is quite different. Honey is also used in some cough syrups. However, it is not an alternative to standard antibiotics.

There is a danger that people listening to this Mufti will just drink honey when they need real antibiotics. He should have explained that people should follow the doctor's advice.

I know two people who gave up the medicines prescribed by doctors in favour of the imam's advice and paid a heavy price. There may be more.

7. Treatment with light

An imam (London E11) told me how it was possible to cure diseases by "light rays". He went into some detail. I asked him how he knew this. He said that he read it in a "book". What he said had no scientific backing.

8. Treatment for cancer

When the cancer patient is sleeping, whisper in his ear: "Dear cancer, you have been living in this body for long, go and find some other body." Cancer will be cured. I asked the imam: "How do you know this?" His answer was: "I read it in a book."

9. Treatment of Corona 2020/2021

Some imams said: "Chant this, chant that 100 times, 300 times, etc., Corona will go. To start, there is no 'Corona'. It is a big conspiracy to destroy Islam and the Muslim way of life."

10. An Imam's Verdict

All diseases are the result of "Possession by Evil Spirits" regardless of whatever aetiology is given in the medical books.

****

With due respect, why do our imams and muftis (from the Indian subcontinent) discuss medical issues when they have no knowledge? My guess is that it is their 'Ego'. Among Asians, the medical profession is regarded as "The highest". It is as if imams feel the need to 'prove' they have some sort of medical knowledge, as they, themselves, are not doctors.

In chapter two, the imam told me: "You are a doctor of medicine, I am a doctor of religion." He had no PhD. His ego was obvious.

Chapter Seventeen
Is the Quran a Pessimistic Book?

Sometimes there is a 'lull' in the operation theatres for various reasons, e.g., staff shortage, waiting for the instruments, or 'a' particular drug not available, equipment coming from another hospital, patient not ready to come to theatres etc. When this happens, we do not have anything to do.

On one of such days, we were chatting in the coffee room in the theatres. One of my non-Muslim colleagues told me that he browsed through the Quran and found it to be a pessimistic book. It is always talking about death, destruction (on/before the Day of Judgment), brutal punishment for crimes in this world and severe punishment in the hereafter, etc. It gives a picture that it is not worth living this life.

I told him that he only browsed through the Quran, that too the translation. It should be read properly. For the full understanding of any verse/chapter, attention should be paid to the accuracy of the translation, the context, the background, any historical event, culture, and customs at the time of its revelation, any phrases of the Arabic language at the time of revelation, and what else has been said about the same topic in other chapters of the Quran.

I gave him a few examples like chapter 4, verse 34. One translation of this verse from an Indian scholar is, "Man is the master, and the women are the slave". Yet the other translation of the same verse from an Arab scholar is, "Man is the breadwinner and protector of women."

My colleague was a junior doctor studying for his exams. I told him, "If you do not study for your exam, you will fail", then I asked him, "is this a pessimistic statement or a realistic statement?" He said it is a real statement. I told him that the Quran and other heavenly books are real books. The Quran in Surah 90, verse 10, says, "…*and We have shown him, meaning Man, both ways, i.e., right and wrong ways, ways of good and evil…*" Then the Quran mentions the consequences of following each way. This is a real statement and not pessimistic.

However, some of the sermons and speeches I have heard (Asian speakers) do give this sort of gloomy picture and the speakers justify this by various verses of the Quran. They try to create 'fear' in the audience's mind so that they would follow the Islamic way of life. They do not mention the positive points, i.e., all the good things you get in the hereafter if you have followed the Islamic principles in your worldly life.

****

On another occasion, I was in the coffee room with other colleagues. There were two junior doctors in the room as well, Ram Gopal (Hindu) and Malik Husain (Muslim) (not the real names). I always encourage the juniors to study and pass the exams.

I asked Ram Gopal about his studies and exams. He said that he was studying hard, and his exam was next month. I asked the same question to Malik Husain. He looked at me for a few seconds and said in Urdu, "Why should I study? After all, one day, I am going to die anyway." Malik Husain may have been under the influence of such so-called 'scholars' who have this pessimistic view. They do not understand Islam. I personally know some of them who say to their followers: "Work for this world as much as you are likely to live here. Work for the hereafter as much as you would live there."

****

A few days ago, I was watching a speech from an Asian scholar on YouTube. This so-called scholar had a perfect appearance of a Muslim religious person. In summary, the 'scholar' said that the salvation for Muslims is to "give up" the world. This is completely against the teaching of the Quran. Giving up the world is condemned in the Quran, Surah: 57, Verse: 27. It is also condemned in the Prophet's sayings. When you read the life of the Prophet, you see that he was a practical man and took full part in worldly affairs. In Madinah, he established the first welfare state in the world. He never said, "Why should I do this or that? One day I am going to die anyway." In surah 62, Verse 10, Allah says to the believers: "*When you finish the Friday prayer, spread out on the earth and look for Allah's bounties.*", meaning, get on with your work.

In Hyderabad, India, and even in the UK, I have come across people from a Muslim religious group who go around knocking on every Muslim's door, saying the same thing again and again. Their message is that this life is not worth living; come with us in the path of Allah. They distracted quite a few young Muslim men from their studies. Some of these young men completely gave up their careers.

All the heavenly books are 'Realistic', none are pessimistic.

Chapter Eighteen
MY GP Friend: This Happened
in the Mid-70s

I had a Muslim GP friend in the north of England. He belonged to a particular group of Muslims who go around preaching Islam to Muslims. They do have some good points (which a Muslim can easily find by studying the Quran), but overall, they are not of my type.

a) This friend of mine, call him "A", once wanted to go on holiday. He asked me if I knew another GP who could do his surgery while "A" goes on holiday. I knew another GP, Dr M, who was looking for some work. I told Dr M to get in touch with A. They got in touch with each other, and M agreed to do the locum work for A.

To get used to the place, people, staff and the patients, M went to A's place a few days earlier and did some surgery sessions with A.

After completing his locum work, M came back to London. I asked him how the work was. M told me that he had never seen a GP like A and he would never work for him. I asked him why and he explained:

Whenever a non-Muslim female patient came to A's surgery, A would look at her, talk to her, examine her, and write the prescription. However, when a Muslim female patient came to the surgery, A would turn away his face from her, just ask her about her symptoms and write a prescription, and hand it over to her without looking at her. M was expected to do the same. This is the reason why M said he would never do A's surgery again. The most surprising thing was that the Muslim female patients were very happy with Dr A, saying that he was so pious that he did not look at "other women". As I was not the direct witness to Dr A's behaviour, I could not have reported it to the General Medical Council.

I asked M to do so, and he said that both A and his patients would deny such practice.

b) Benefits of doing regular prayers. I have mentioned it somewhere, but I will repeat it.

Once I was a guest in A's house. We both came back from the mosque after the night prayer. A started telling me about the benefits of doing regular prayers. He said, "On the day of resurrection, all the beautiful women (hoors) would be brought in front of men. These beautiful women would have seventy layers of clothes on them. Those men, who did their regular prayers in this world, would get such power in their sight that despite hoors having seventy layers of clothes, these men would be able to see the hoors naked."

I asked him who told him this rubbish. He said, "the Ameer, i.e., leader, of his particular group", the preaching party.

I told this whole story to other imams. They all declared this as total nonsense.

c) Hajj, 17 times: This Dr A, went to Hajj, for the first time in his life. Hajj is a daunting task, physically, because of the number of people, in millions, doing certain rituals at the same time and in the same place. Almost everyone who goes to Hajj has one or more stories to tell about the problems and incidences they encounter while performing Hajj.

When Dr A came back from Hajj, I asked him about his experience. I was expecting that he would talk about various problems he would have had, especially because it was his first time. His answer was that he had absolutely no problems at all. This was very surprising. I asked him how that happened. He said:

"In my group, there was one person who had done Hajj seventeen times. He knew all the pitfalls and how to avoid them. He made my Hajj very easy."

I asked Dr A about this person who did Hajj seventeen times. I asked if this person was hired by some Hajj organisers, or was he the leader of some group/s to help people there, etc. Dr A said that there was nothing like that. This person had no job for years, was surviving on social security and had nothing else to do but to go on Hajj. He was not a disabled person either.

To me, this is a complete waste of money. Hajj is obligatory once in a lifetime for those who can afford it financially. Doing Hajj seventeen times, paid by the taxpayer's money, is a total waste. He could have used the same money to do better jobs like helping those in need.

Some people regard social security as their right. I have also heard claims like, "Social security is our right; it is our money, stolen by British people when they were ruling over the Indian subcontinent."

These are all senseless justifications for creating a feel-good factor in them that they are not doing anything wrong.

d) Islamic upbringing of children.

This GP friend of mine Dr A, regarded me as a junior person when it came to the knowledge of Islam (although we are of the same age and were classmates in the medical school in Hyderabad, India). This is because he belongs to a particular group of Muslims who go around preaching Islam to Muslims only. He used to teach me various Islamic practices and benefits of following Islam, like the benefits of doing regular prayers, which I mentioned above.

Once, this GP friend told me that to keep the children's Islamic upbringing up to date, it is essential to beat them once a month. This is total non-sense.

PS: I am not in touch with this GP friend. I do not know if he is alive or dead. I do not know the whereabouts of my doctor friend who did the locum for this GP on my request. This was the one and only case of this kind I know. A vast majority of doctors, regardless of their religion, are honest, sincere, and conscious about their duties.

Chapter Nineteen
Some More (39) Short Stories
(All are Strange but True)

1). Hypocrisy and blind belief

All the Asian scholars/maulvis I have listened to (and read) say that music is *haram (forbidden)* in Islam.

Among the audience, in any religious gathering, there are mainly two types of people. **A)**. Those who nod their heads in agreement blindly believe in everything the speaker says and follow the advice without question. They do so for everything they hear/ read in the name of Islam. These are the **blind believers. B)**. Those who nod their heads, "Yes Sir, Yes Sir", just to agree, and do not believe and do not follow the advice. They are the **hypocrites**.

****

With regard to music: 1. This word is not mentioned in the Quran. 2. Those Asian scholars who believe in music being haram quote verses from chapter 31, V 6 and chapter 41, V 26. However, Arab scholars, like A. Yusuf Ali and Adil Silahi do not see these verses in favour of music being haram. If you read these verses with an independent, unbiased, un-influenced mind, you will come to the same conclusion as the above two.

In the book "Our Dialogue", volume *IV, page 92 and 93 (published by apkar PK, Karachi, Pakistan)*, the author, Adil Silahi, an Arab, discusses this issue in detail, with the conclusion that music is not haram as the Asian scholars say.

****

All the psychologists, including Muslim psychologists, say that music has a positive effect on mind and memory. However, this approach i.e., music being permitted, comes with certain limitations, which you will know if you know the Quran well.

****

Other examples of hypocrisy. I know some religious people who in public say that interest is haram and yet take mortgages and students loans. Others say that watching TV is haram, and they have TVs in their homes.

I have given many examples of blind believes in this book, including a person, my close relative, who removed the pictures of his family members in his house because his teacher told him that photography was forbidden in Islam. It is not universally accepted that photography is forbidden in Islam.

With a little bit of courage, we can overcome the hypocrisy and with a little bit of thinking, we can get rid of this kind of blind beliefs.

2). My encounter with…

It is my belief that one should be aware of his surroundings and what is going on in his locality, in his town/city/ country and even internationally, as this affects him or his family, directly or indirectly in a positive or negative way.

When I had an encounter with the prostitutes (chapter 1:42), I kept thinking for few days as to why these girls end up like this.

Then there was a series of documentaries on TV about them, so I watched the series. Some interesting points were:

They showed three girls in that profession, who in day light were, a medical student, an economics student, and a law student. They justified their 'profession' by saying, "Oh, it is fun, and it gives me some pocket money." "Oh, I have been doing this since my teens." "Oh, it is a way of socialisation; I get to meet new people all the time." I am not discussing the right or wrong of what they were doing, but I found it interesting; how one can justify his/her actions.

They showed another girl who appeared with her husband. The husband was happy that the wife was bringing home, a good amount of money. Sometimes, the husband dropped his wife at the client's house and waited outside till the session finished.

The interviewer asked her: "Do you feel any difference between your clients and your husband?" Her answer was, "Yes, when I am with my clients, I am having sex, without any feelings, without any emotions, it is a job. However, when I am with my husband, I am making love, with feelings and emotions."

In the Daily Mail on Wednesday 18 April 2018, a similar story appeared. This was taken from the Victoria Derbyshire show, BBC 2, shown on 17 April 2018. The girl wanted to pay off her student loan, so she came into the profession.

These girls reminded me of my work as a doctor in India. I have seen so many cases of sexually transmitted diseases like gonorrhoea, primary, secondary, and even tertiary syphilis, both in women as well as in their clients. Here, in the UK I have not come across any such cases. None of my patients, who came for surgery, had any of the above diseases, but I have come across HIV positive and Aids patients.

Regardless of the rights or wrongs of their job, these women get a good health check-up in this country which is one of the many good things this country offers to its citizens.

3). …but he is a Muslim.

I was new in the hospital, London E13. Not many people knew me nor my work except the theatre manager, an English man.

I was in the kitchen of the operation theatres, making a cup of coffee for myself, when I overheard, in the adjacent sitting room, someone asking the theatre manager how I was to work with. The manager said: "He is very nice, polite, very efficient, very punctual, very organised, methodical, very conscious about his work etc., etc.…but he is a Muslim."

Even to date, I do not know what this meant.

4). Are you hiding any bombs?

I was having a loft conversion in my house in London. The architect, an old English gentleman, came to see the loft. As he was about to go up, I told him to take his shoes off. He asked me "why?" And I told him that in our house, as a Muslim, outside shoes were allowed up to a certain point.

As he was about to enter the loft, he turned round and asked me: "you are Muslim, yes?" I said: "yes". Then he said: "How many bombs are you hiding in the loft?"

I told him that I was letting him go this time, but any more comments like this, and I was cancelling the contract.

A Few people do something wrong and the whole community gets the blame.

I suppose this is human nature. Muslims are not the only ones targeted.

A Sri-Lankan lady colleague of mine is married to an Irishman. She told me that when she told her parents about "him", they said, "Are you marrying an Irishman? They are all IRA terrorists."

Unfortunately, people of African and Central American origin have a negative image as well. I have many colleagues from these countries, and I found them to be very nice people.

Recently (2020), the death of George Floyd in the US started a protest, "Black lives matter." Discrimination is part of human nature; only with education and by following your religious teachings, you can eradicate it.

5). Friday sermon that spoiled my prayer.

In the multi-faith/quiet room of my hospital in London, we hold regular Friday prayers. This Friday sermon was delivered by a known imam in my hospital.

In his sermon, he mentioned a story in which a woman was completely naked in a one-bedroom desert house. Instead of a proper door at the entrance of the house, there was only a curtain hanging. Each time the wind blew, the curtain was lifting, and any outsider could see the naked woman. Then he mentioned a young man who was passing by, and he was distracted, then controlled himself; then distracted, then controlled himself etc. The imam used the word "naked woman" five times during his sermon.

When you are being told a story, you start imagining the scenes in the story. The same thing happened here as well. I do not know about others; it is very easy for me to imagine a naked woman because I worked in the operation theatres for many years and during this time, there was hardly a day when I had not seen a naked woman.

The result was that this sermon spoiled my Friday prayer.

People, who bring sex and women into their speeches in the mosques, probably get some sort of sexual gratification. I could see the pleasure on the imam's face each time he mentioned the word "naked woman."

Is this Islam?

An outside speaker in my local mosque was telling the story of King Solomon having sex with his nine hundred wives in one night. I could see the pleasure on his face while he was telling the story.

The same pleasure was seen on the face of another imam, who was telling the story of Moses running naked after a stone ran away with his clothes.

Is this Islam? Is this what they learn in religious schools?

6). Mission accomplished…come back home.

I have always believed that God sends some men/women to this world to accomplish certain job/s. Once the job is accomplished, He calls them back 'home'…the real home of all of us. Below are some examples:

a) Surah 5, verse 3: "…Today We have perfected your deen (religion), completed all our favours to you, and agreed for Islam to be your deen."

This was the last verse to be revealed. All the companions were very happy, but Abu-Bakar, the 1st Khalif (R.A.), was sad. When asked why was he sad? He replied, "This verse means mission accomplished; it is time for the Prophet (PBUH) to go home."

The Prophet died within three months of this verse being revealed.

Mission accomplished…come back home.

Of course, this is the best example, but at ordinary levels, one can find examples of "mission accomplished, come home." Below are two examples:

b) Henry Grey.

As a first-year medical student in Hyderabad, India, I was very impressed by the "A textbook of human anatomy" by Henry Grey. This is the most comprehensive, most accurate book ever written on human anatomy. Millions of medical students and people of allied professions benefitted by this book. The anatomy for all the surgical procedures, procedures in intensive care units and other procedures on the human body originate from this book. Although later, other people have written books on human anatomy, Grey's anatomy is the most comprehensive.

Henry Grey started writing this book at the age of 24. He spent most of his time in the dissection hall. It took him ten years to complete this book. Once the book was complete, at the age of 34, he died.

Mission accomplished…Come back home.

c) Sisters got married.

In the early 1950s, my eldest brother had a classmate called Mohi Uddin. He came from a poor family. His mother was a widow, and he had two elder sisters.

Mohi Uddin's mother was always worried about how she was going to see her two daughters getting married. There was no money. In the Indian sub-continent, in those days and even now, a daughter's wedding is a huge burden on the parents.

Mohi Uddin graduated and managed to find a job, which was enough to get by but not enough to save for his sisters' marriages.

On his first day to start the job, Mohi Uddin set out from his house, got a bus to go to the workplace. The bus had an accident. Out of 40 passengers on the bus, Mohi Uddin was the only one who died.

As he was a young man with a bright and long future, the compensation his mother got from the bus company was enough to see her two daughters getting married. The mother always used to say, "my son died so that my daughters could get married." Mohi Uddin was sent to this world just for that.

Mission accomplished...Come back home.

I am sure there are many examples like these.

7). When is Christmas? When is Diwali? When is Eid?

The answer to the first two events is clear. Well, in advance, we can say when Christmas and Diwali are. When it comes to Eid, only one night before, we can say that too, not for sure for the entire country. This has been a laughing matter for years.

Like every year, this year also, some places in southern England celebrated Eid one day after the majority of Muslims celebrated Eid. Did the new moon appear twice in England?

Last year I heard the funniest joke. In Croydon, living in the same house, under the same roof, the father celebrated Eid because Ramadhan had ended for him, whereas the son was fasting because it was the 30th of Ramadhan for him. There were two different dates in the same place at the same time. Is this the miracle of the 21st century? Only Muslims are capable of performing such miracles.

Just yesterday, 5 July 2017, I saw a cartoon on my phone, in which the devil is saying, "with all these different dates of Eid, when am I coming out of prison?"

The solution to this problem is observatory. I have said this to our local imams many times, but each time I got only one answer i.e., "it is against Sunnah." Going by the observatory, we can say well in advance, when the new moon would be. But as usual, Muslims are far behind in science and in taking advantage of any scientific achievements. Living in 21st century western world, they want to live a life of 6th century Saudi Arabia. Our imams, religious leaders and members of the moon sighting committee need to consider these points seriously.

By following the observatory, we are not breaking the basic rule of Sunnah that the new Islamic month starts with the birth of a new moon. One of the imam's comments to this was: "Oh no, we have to see the moon with naked eyes." In the northern hemisphere, way away from the equator, with clouds on the horizon most of the time, how often can you see the new moon?

One question I asked imams, for which they have no satisfactory answer, is: "If you are so anti-observatory, why do you and each mosque publish the entire year's prayer timings, well in advance, based on the observatory? When it is time for Maghreb prayer (prayer soon after sun set), do you go out and see if the sun has set? Of course not; you rely on the sunset time given by the observatory. Why are you following the observatory now? When it is Fajar prayer time, which must be done before sunrise, do you go out and see if the sun is rising? Of course not; you rely on the sunrise time given by the observatory. If you are following the observatory every day, twice a day, for 365 days, why not follow it for the dates of the new moon?

It will make life easy, especially for the working population in the western world. For example, if you want to take time off for Eid, you will be able to tell your employer well in advance rather than phoning 'off sick' in the morning. If you phone off sick in the morning, you are starting your Eid with a lie. The imams will not understand this because, unlike the mainstream, their 'job' is in the mosques only. They do not have any 'scheduled surgical operations, scheduled interviews, scheduled meetings, scheduled programmes etc.' Life is easy for them.

We had a Muslim nurse in our operation theatres. She used to go off sick in Ramadhan very frequently so that she could fast. She used to ring in the morning and say that she was off sick for that day. Everyone knew that it was a lie. It was so difficult to find a replacement for her at such short notice. It was a common say in the theatres: "Ramadhan is approaching. It is time for Miss Z to go off sick."

One day I told "Z" that she should not do this. Everyone knew that she lied. She said: "Oh. Everyone does this." Although it was not the right answer, it was better than saying: "It is OK to cheat whites." (See chapter 9 on it is OK to cheat whites.)

The main difficulty nurse Z had was that she did not know when Ramadhan would be starting until the night before. There was not enough time to give notice of absence. Here, she was right. This problem could be solved if Muslims follow the observatory for the new moon. Then we would know, for sure, when an Islamic month would start.

8). Islamic calendar...*unworkable*.

Somebody I know is very keen on everything 'Islamic'. He says that we should not follow the Christian calendar (Solar calendar) but follow the Islamic calendar (Lunar months calendar). I told him that it would not work unless we bring a fundamental change. This change will not compromise the basic principle. I gave him two examples of why it would not work in its present state, i.e., the 1st day of the next lunar month will be known only a night before.

Example: 1. You are the director of a company, or a hospital manager, or you run your own business based in London. You have some vacancies in your organisation, and you advertise for these posts.

Someone from Leeds applies for the job. Following the Islamic calendar, you ask him to come to London for an interview on the 10th of Shawwal, an Islamic month. On that day, i.e., 10th of Shawwal, you wait and wait for this candidate and he does not turn up. You ring him and ask why he did not come? His answer is. "you asked me to come on the 10th of Shawwal and today it is the 9th of Shawwal." You say, "No, it is the 10th of Shawwal in London." He says, "but it is 9th of Shawwal in Leeds."

Here is the problem. While 10th March is 10th March throughout the country and in the world, the 10th of Shawwal in London is 9th of Shawwal in Leeds.

This problem is very easy to sort out if we follow the observatory, where dates of the new moon are fixed. If we stick to our present behaviour, i.e., living in the 21st-century western world, and people try to follow the 6th century Saudi Arabian way of life, we will never be able to sort out this problem.

By following the observatory, we are not deviating from the Quran (Surah 10, verse 5) but following it in a much better way, to our advantage.

In the above verse, Allah says, "…We have made the moon to be a light (reflected) and measured out stages for it so that you may count the number of years and the time…"

When I discussed this with imams, they say that it is Sunnah to view the new moon with the naked eye. For this, I say that in the 6th century Saudi Arabia, there was no observatory, and the horizon was almost always clear. It was easy to see the new moon. This is not the case in the western world, northern hemisphere, thousands of miles away from the equator, where most of the time, the horizon is not clear. The other question I ask was: "Why do you follow the observatory for the prayer times? For the timings of sunrise and sunset? Why don't you go out each morning and each evening to see if the sun is rising and setting?"

I did not find any answer to my questions.

Example: 2. I am a doctor. I send letters to the patients saying that their operations are due on the 30th of Moharram (an Islamic month) and they should be in the hospital at 7 a.m.

Only on the 29th of Moharram, after the sunset, I discover that "Oh dear, tomorrow is not the 30th of Moharram but 1st of Safar, an Islamic month following Moharram. I have already scheduled other patients for the 1st of Safar; where am I going to accommodate the patients I have scheduled for surgery on the 30th of Moharram? As there is no 30th of Moharram and I discovered this only last night."

This is an unworkable, impractical Islam and it should not be like this if we take advantage of the dates of the new moon from the observatory.

9). What is wrong with your religion?

Why are your women so backward?

I was working in an East London hospital, which was a branch of the main hospital, about five miles away.

I was waiting in the coffee room of this branch hospital for a consultant gynaecologist (Sri Lankan guy).

Around 9:30 a.m., he dashed into the coffee room and, addressing me, shouted in a loud voice:

"What is wrong with your religion? Why are your women so backward?"

I told him: "Calm down Mr R. and tell me why you are so angry?"

The story emerged that when he was ready to come to the branch hospital from the main Hospital, he offered a lift to a Muslim lady doctor, who was a member of his team and was due to come to this branch hospital. The lady doctor refused his offer. He regarded this as an insult. This was the reason for him being so angry and saying that something was wrong with Islam and Muslim women were backward.

If a woman does not accept a lift from another man, it is her free will. This should not be taken as an insult. Women have an extra faculty by which they can sense if a man is safe or not.

Mr R. did not know that a few days earlier, a Muslim male doctor offered a lift to a Hindu lady doctor, and she refused. The Muslim doctor did not mind and made no fuss about the issue.

Mr R. did not know that in Hindu mythology, there is the concept of "Laxman Rekha", which puts certain restrictions on a woman's attitude towards other men. This concept is in other religions as well. In Islam, it is called attitude towards "non-mahram". A non-mahram is a member of the opposite sex who is marriageable to the person but not married to her/him.

Mr R. did not know that a surgical registrar was sacked for misbehaving with his secretary in a situation where the secretary was alone in her office.

I know a consultant physician who also lost his job because of complaints from female lady doctors.

I also know a consultant gynaecologist who is behind bars for misbehaving with his patients.

Mr R's attitude has always been very anti-Muslim. He could not see any Muslim rising in his career. He always used to ask me, "when are you retiring?"

Of course, everyone is not like Mr R. I have some very nice Hindu friends.

In my career and even now, I never differentiated anyone on the basis of his/her religion, cast, colour, nationality or anything like this. I have given very good references to some Hindu doctors because they deserved it. Some of my Hindu patients have written very nice letters of thanks to me for the care I provided them.

Mr R. was not the only anti-Muslim doctor I have come across. There were two lady gynaecologists (one in India, another one in London). They were extremely anti-Muslim too.

To be fair, I know two Muslim doctors; they are very anti-Hindu and anti-Shia.

Prejudice in any form is part of human nature. All religions condemn it. It is a test for every human to see if he/she is fair and unbiased.

10). Doctors' prejudice.

My mind went back to 1971, Osmania Hospital, Hyderabad, India. Among many very good, unbiased doctors in that hospital, there were two doctors, one Hindu and another Muslim, who were very biased. Whenever the Hindu doctor was on call for the night, he admitted all the Hindu patients from E.R. (emergency room), and when the Muslim doctor was on call for the night, he admitted all the Muslim patients from E.R. Patients were admitted to the hospital on the grounds of their religion and not on the grounds of their needs.

These two doctors will have a lot to answer when they will stand in front of God.

Biasness/hatred, racism, ill feelings towards others, etc., are elements of human nature. What happened in Charlottesville, USA, in August 2017 (white supremacist riots) and the slogan "black lives matter" in 2020 after George Floyd's murder are two of many examples. One must suppress these feelings actively as this is not part of any religion.

On BBC Asian radio, in London, I heard about a Sikh who joined the EDL (English Defence League). His reason for joining was that at the time of the partition of India, his father was killed by Muslims. This should not be the grudge to hold against Muslims as many Muslims were killed by Sikhs at that time. That era should be forgotten as a 'bad dream'. It is the fault of our forefathers, and we should not carry the 'revenge feelings' onwards and be biased against each other.

On the 70th anniversary of the creation of Pakistan (14 August 2017) and the independence of India (15 August 2017), the BBC television sent its reporter, Rita Chekrbati, to India and Anita Rani to Pakistan. Their reports contained some old film footage. They were very fair in saying that in Punjab, Hindus and Sikhs killed Muslims and vice versa.

We all can live in peace and harmony if we get rid of such ill feelings. This will be a religious act, regardless of whatever your religion is.

11). What is your caste?

When I was a single man, I got a proposal for marriage through a middleman. This is a typical way of arranging marriages among Asians. This proposal was immediately rejected by the girl's father when he asked me: "What is your caste?" and my answer was: "I do not have a caste. I am a Muslim and in Islam, there is no caste system. God has created all humans "equal". Apparently, this was news to him that God has created everyone equal. He belonged to that part of the Indian subcontinent where the belief is: "God has created two types of people, one who gives orders and another who takes the orders." This was told to me by one of my Punjabi friends, a doctor who belonged to the 1st category (landlords), feudal lords.

Is this Islam? How can they be Muslims when they do not know even the basics of Islam?

Probably, this concept is the very much distorted and misunderstood form of verse 32, Surah 43, which says: "*We raised some of them, i.e., Humans, above the others so that some may employ others in their work.*" This is an important principle to keep worldly affairs running smoothly. In the UK, if everyone is the prime minister, who is going to do other jobs? In the hospitals, if everyone is a consultant, who is going to do the junior doctors job? This does not mean that one is a superior human being to the other. In the eyes of God, one who is more pious is more honourable and respectable than the one who is not/less pious, Surah 49, verse 13.

The majority of Asians do not read (study) the Quran on a regular basis. Those who do, do so for rewards only, therefore, do not know the meaning of what they are reading. A smaller portion does read the meanings, but in translations only, in their own languages. Not all translations and explanations give the correct meanings, as they depend on the translator's views, interpretation, knowledge of Arabic language and knowledge of his own language in which he is translating the Quran and other factors.

It is said that when Dr Maurice Bucaille, a French doctor, asked King Faisal of Saudi Arabia as to which translation of the Quran should he read. King Faisal told him to learn Arabic and then read the actual text.

Of course, it is not easy for everyone to learn Arabic and read the Quran in Arabic. Translation gives the reader the basic message of the Quran, i.e., Oneness of God, belief in His messengers, Belief in accountability and good deeds.

To go into more details and for the Quran to touch your heart, you need to read it in Arabic.

12). We are Sayyeds.

In Arabic, Sayyed simply means "Mr". The term Sayyeds (men) and Sayyadats (ladies) are used in general conversations. For example, if you travel in Saudi Arabian Airline or any other Arab Airline, the pilot, when making an announcement, starts with: "Sayyadats and Sayyeds", meaning Ladies and Gentlemen. In Arab countries, even toilets are labelled as "Sayyed" and "Sayyadats", meaning toilets for men and ladies.

I have worked in Saudi Arabia and I have come across many Arab doctors in the UK. I have not come across a single Arab whose name starts with Sayyed.

However, when Islam reached the Indian Subcontinent and got mixed up and muddled up with local traditions and culture, things changed quite a bit. Now, Sayyeds, in the Indian subcontinent are regarded as the direct descendants of the Prophet Muhammed (PBUH) and, therefore, automatically, have a higher position in the Muslim community. They are like "Brahmins" in the Hindu religion who are supposed to be the custodian of the religion.

In Islam (and other religions), the law is the same for all. Nobody is above the law.

The Prophet (PBUH) said: "Even if my daughter Fatima steals anything, the punishment is the same as for anyone else who steals."

Verses 44-47 of the Surah 69 say clearly that even the Prophet is not above the law.

Surah 49, verse 10 clearly says: "All believers are brothers to each other."

In his last sermon, on the mount Arafat, the Prophet (PBUH) said, among many things:

"Arabs have no superiority over non-Arabs; Whites have no superiority over blacks."

The Sayyeds in the Indian subcontinent regards themselves as of the highest caste, and therefore would not marry in families who are not Sayyed.

This can and has caused problems:

a) In Hyderabad.

There was a Sayyed family with two daughters. When the girls grew up, some marriage proposals came for them from non-Sayyed families. The boys were well educated and had jobs. However, they were immediately rejected by the father, who was adamant that the girls would marry only in a Sayyed family. The time passed. No suitable Sayyed could be found. The girls were getting old and had their 'needs'. One day, it was found that they ran away from home with some men.

b) In London.

There was a Sayyed family with one daughter who was a highly qualified, professional person, with a good job, good pay and was very pretty as well. Marriage proposals came from non-Sayyeds and were rejected by the father. He was adamant that the girl must marry a Sayyed. At last, the father found a man from the Indian subcontinent who was a Sayyed, totally uneducated and had never left his country before. He was brought here, in London, the girl got married to him and the marriage ended up in divorce within six months. The reasons were: the man was already married in his country of origin, had a wife and two children, had quite a few bad habits, including some of his demands towards his wife to act, which no decent woman would do.

There must be many more cases like these, all because one human being considers himself superior to others.

c) When I was working in Harrogate General Hospital, Yorkshire, I had a colleague who was a Sayyed, from Pakistan. He was well known for his 'Gallivanting' activities.

d) There are many Asian Muslim prisoners in European jails. There are Sayyeds among them.

e) Some Sayyeds in India (I do not know about Pakistan) claim that they are the masters of non-Sayyeds and can treat them however they like.

f) Some Sayyeds can give a person a guarantee of paradise, written on a piece of paper, to be buried with that person.

The most astonishing thing I found that common people in India believe in the superiority of Sayyeds. As I have said before: "It is very easy to fool people in the name of religion."

For more on this topic, see "Islamic way of thinking" by Adil Salahi, 3rd edition, December 2000, pages 442-447. The book is in Urdu; I have translated the name into English.

13). Brides of the Quran.

A few years ago, this was the title of a TV programme.

The programme showed that some 'elite' Muslim families in the Indian Subcontinent (an Asian Muslim country) were marrying their daughters to the Quran. The idea was to keep the family's wealth within the family. These brides of the Quran, to full fill their needs, had illegal relationships.

Marriage is a psychological, physiological, and physical need for both men and women. These needs must be fulfilled in proper, legal ways; otherwise, the 'needy' people start fulfilling their needs in illegal ways.

This reminds me of the **Middle East.**

Many people from the Indian subcontinent go to the Middle Eastern countries to build a better life back at home. Many of them leave their families back at home either to save money or for the education of children. The wives are left behind with husbands visiting once every six months or once a year. There have been cases where wives, to fulfil their physical needs, started having relationships with other men.

This also may be a problem for people working on the ships. They are away on ships for six months or more, leaving their wives behind. In one of the hospitals I worked at, there was a nurse whose husband used to be away, on his ship, coming home once every six months. There were a lot of rumours about this girl.

This reminds me of an incident at the time of Umar (R.A.). He was on a night round and found a woman singing in the memory of her husband, who was away in an expedition (army). Umar realised that sending men away for a long time was not the right thing to do. Consulting his wife and other women, he made a necessary reduction in the period for which men should be away from their families.

A lonely woman, without the chaperon of a man, is easy prey for opportunistic men. No matter how much she would resist, she would give up at some point because she also has her natural needs. You cannot fight nature. Most of these needs are fulfilled from 'within the family' resources where there are free and unsuspected movements of the family members. I personally know some incidences.

14). The interest money, Muslim Aid, a Bombay businessman.

With the complexity of modern finances, especially in the western world, it is impossible to avoid interest money indirectly. For example, the local councils in England are given their annual budget at the beginning of the financial year. The councils put this money in the highest 'interest-paying' banks.

So, if you are an employee in a council, part of your monthly payment is coming from the interest money which the council is getting from the bank. You cannot avoid it.

There are many examples like this, both in the public and private sectors.

I am a regular donor to Muslim Aid. A few years back, it sent me a letter saying that whatever "Interest" you get on your savings in the banks and building societies, give it to Muslim Aid. It has taken a Fatwa that it is OK to use this money for the benefits of the needy.

In 2017, during Ramadhan, I attended a talk on Zakat given by the National Zakat Foundation at Redbridge Islamic Centre, East London (Essex). They also said that any interest you get on your savings must be given to charity.

It is important to note that this 'giving away of interest money' is in addition to the Zakat due on your wealth. It should **NEVER** be a part of your zakat.

This reminds me of an incident that was told to me by my uncle.

In the 1950s (when I was a child), there was a very successful Muslim businessman in Bombay. He had large sums of money left in his account in the bank. The interest kept mounting on this money. When the sum became very large, the bank asked the businessman what to do with this money. The businessman said: "I am a Muslim, in Islam interest is haram, and therefore you do whatever you want to do with this money." Later, he came to know that the bank had used it for very un-Islamic purposes.

In my view, the businessman should have asked the bank what it was going to do with that money and then decide whether to leave the money with the bank or not. He simply and rigidly followed the rule: "Interest is haram; therefore, I am nothing to do with it."

Sometimes, depending on the circumstances, you may have to bend the rules. This 'bending of the rule' applies only for that time, for that reason. The fundamental principle stays the same.

Student loans are another example where the rules need to be bent, for a very good purpose; otherwise, the vast majority of Muslim children will not go to university.

Even in today's London, I have seen bending of the rules, for example:

The rule (according to the imam of my local mosque) says that for any prescribed prayer, there should not be two congregational prayers in a mosque, i.e., for example, for midday prayer, there should be only one congregational prayer. Similarly, there should not be two Friday prayers or Eid prayers in the same mosque. However, I have seen in my local mosques, on Good Friday, they hold two or more congregational prayers. The same is for Eid prayers as well.

Sometimes, your own personal circumstances are such that you must bend the rules. Your intention must be clean, when the circumstances revert, you must go back to normal practice.

15). Not a bad deal at all.

In the mid-1970s, I was working in a London hospital. On a Friday afternoon, I was in the operation theatres with an assistant lady doctor, J. She was from Durban, South Africa. Around 2:30 p.m., J asked me if she could leave early, around 3 p.m. I said OK and she left at 3 p.m.

On the following Monday, J was supposed to be with me in the morning. She did not turn up. Around 10 a.m., she rang me saying that she was going to be another one hour late. She came to the operation theatres at 11 a.m.

I asked her if everything was OK with her as she left early on Friday and came late on Monday. She said that she went to Durban, South Africa, for the weekend. I said, "it must have been very expensive for you to go there, just for a weekend." She said that she paid only £10 for the return flight, as her mother was an air hostess in the South African airline. Employees of airlines get many concessions. Then she said, "it was **not a bad deal at all**". I agreed.

Food for thought: If the average life span of a person is taken as 80 years, then the first ten to fifteen years are spent in childhood, with little understanding of the world and purpose of our life. In the remaining time, about 20 years are lost in sleep. This leaves around 45 years. If we follow God's commands in these

45 years, then we are bound to get an eternal life of peace, comfort, luxury, and no worries. It is **not a bad deal at all.**

16). "Move away, angels are coming." Angels bring Coke and sandwiches.

I have heard this from two reliable sources. I was not present to witness these two incidences.

This is about a well-known scholar of Islam, with millions of followers around the world. For the purpose of writing, I call him Dr T.

a) A person died. At his funeral, Dr T was present and was the main lead in all the prayers etc. After the burial, he told his followers, "Move away, move away, because angels are coming, and I am going to talk to them." The followers, the *blind believers*, moved away. Dr T was standing near the grave. He looked up in the sky, uttered few words which no one could hear and that was the end of his conversation with the angels.

The funniest thing was all the followers believed that he did speak to the angles.

b) In another incident, Dr T went to Mecca for the pilgrimage and decided to climb to the cave of Hira, which is at the top of the mountain. It is a fairly high mountain. As he was tired and needed a drink, he looked at the sky, prayed for a drink and the angels brought him cans of Coke in a tray. As he was coming down from the cave, he was hungry and again, his prayers were answered, and the angels brought him some sandwiches.

BBC News: 29-08-2017. A holy man in Punchcola, Haryana, India, named Gourmet Ram, Rahim Singh, who also has millions of followers and land and property in India, has been jailed for 20 years for raping two women, his devotees. There have been riots, and many people died because the followers refused to believe that the guru could do anything like this.

Again, I will say the same thing, which I have said before: "It is very easy to fool people in the name of religion, whether it is Islam or any other religion."

17). Prayers during working hours.

a) In Muslim countries, time is given for this. Be thankful to the management for this facility, but do not abuse it. Prayers, according to the degree of importance, are of four types. MSCm is the short form for these degrees. M=Must be done (Obligatory prayers), S=should be done (Wajib prayers, like Witer and sunnat-e-mou-akkidah), C=can be done and m=may be done. Only obligatory prayers are "must". To do additional voluntary prayers depends on the nature of your work. Your work should not be affected by these prayers. Many times, in Saudi Arabia, I did my "obligatory" prayers in the coffee room of the operation theatres because I had surgical lists to start. I did not have time to go to the mosque and I did not have time for voluntary prayers either. At least, I was satisfied that I was doing my work honestly and sincerely and my pay was all halal (genuine/legal).

Those who did go to the mosque came back very late. We had to turn a 'blind eye' to them. There were many non-Muslim doctors who started work in time, thus the service ran smoothly.

b) In the western world, performing prayers during working hours may be a problem. These days, almost every workplace has a 'multi-faith' room. This is a great facility given by the caring and considerate management. However, 'time' may be a problem. While working in the hospitals in the UK I have always done my prayers at a time when my patients were in 'no danger'. On some occasions, when I was needed urgently, I interrupted my prayers and attended the emergency.

Doctor's action:

I do not believe that 'this' doctor's actions were right who never answered his bleep on Fridays between 1 p.m. and 2 p.m., no matter how urgently he was needed. Ultimately, he was brought to the disciplinary committee and was given a verbal warning. Your work, for which you are paid, comes first. This doctor followed the rules blindly, i.e., prayers must be done ON time, without understanding them.

18). Punishment for your sins.

I personally did not attend this Friday prayer sermon in a London E11 mosque. Someone who did attend asked me the validity of what was said.

The imam, from the Indian sub-continent, qualified in a religious school there, said quite a few things about sins and punishment. Then he said: "If Allah wants to punish someone for his sins, He gives him daughters. For example, Jews have done and still do, lot of mischievous things; therefore, Allah punishes them by giving them more girls."

My comment: "This is complete nonsense. Did that Imam forget that our Prophet (PBUH) had four daughters and two sons?

Since it is not possible for all Muslims to study the Quran in-depth and understand it very well, Allah says in the Quran that "a" group of Muslims need to study the religion, understand it. and then teach others; Surah 9, verse 122. This is how "madrassahs" (religious schools) came into existence. This is fine. This is what the four great imams and their students did. They did a great job. There is absolutely nothing wrong with their teachings, although there are differences of opinions on minor issues. None of them violated the fundamental principles of Islam.

However, the question which comes to my mind is that what do we do with 'some' of the present day's imams like the one above? Or the like those in other chapters of this book, i.e., MRI and Tiger, Professor of Physics and 666, Who, Why, When What Where, Jinns did it and many more. They are all qualified imams from religious schools.

This is the reason I encourage everyone to study the Quran and not to have a blind belief in what you hear or read.

Doctors and other professionals have regulatory bodies which keep an eye on them. They are supposed to have annual appraisals, keep up with CPDs (Continuous Professional Developments), regular training and revalidations for doctors.

There is no such thing as regulatory bodies for imams and muftis. Once qualified from a religious school, they are free for life to say whatever they want to say. There is no such thing as CPD or Accreditation or Annual Appraisal for them. In most of the Middle Eastern countries, Friday sermons are given to them, approved by the governments. Imams cannot say anything other than what is already written in the sermons. This may be politically motivated, but at least these sermons do not contain things like what I have written above and in other chapters of this book or statements like: "*We have got nothing to do with science and technology. We have come in this world to keep saying...Allah, Allah.*" This was said in the sermon on a Friday in my local mosque.

I think that a regulatory body should be formed by sensible, educated scholars of Islam. Imams should be interviewed once a year and their views on various issues, including current affairs, should be known. If needed, they should be educated to get rid of silly beliefs like if you are a bad guy, you will get more daughters. In 2020, there are imams who believe that Coronavirus is a hoax, a conspiracy to destroy Islam and the Muslim way of life.

I have great respect for our imams, religious leaders, and scholars. They do a great job; they lead the nation. They meet the spiritual and religious needs of society.

However, I do not have a blind belief in them. If they say/ write something which is not right in my view, I need to say so, otherwise, I may be accountable for not speaking out.

19). Twenty evil plots under every hair.

I read this story on YouTube. I do not know if it is true or not. The story is as follows:

A Muslim man (Asian) went to the mosque to listen to the sermon by the maulvi sahib.

During his speech, the speaker said that every woman is evil; every woman hides 20 evil plots under each hair on her head.

The man came home and shaved his wife's head completely.

I think this is just a made-up story. However, this reminded me of another conversation between me and other maulvi years ago, when I was in India.

The maulvi told me that women are evil; it is in her nature. I asked him what the proof was that women are evil. He said, "It is in the Quran, I am 100% sure". "Where?" I asked. He said it is written in the story of Prophet Yusuf (Joseph). I knew the story very well. He was referring to Surah 12, verse 28. I told him that before saying anything about the Quran, that too so categorically, think twice, and go into the details.

The story is that Prophet Yusuf was seduced by the wife of the Lord of Egypt (Aziz). She made excuses, but Aziz found out the truth and then said, "Surely, it is a plot of you women. Certainly, mighty is the plot of you, women."

I told this maulvi sahib that these are the words of Aziz and not the words of Allah. Allah is simply quoting Aziz's words. Just because you quote someone's words does not mean that you agree with what that person is saying. I gave him another example: In another place in the Quran, Surah 79, verse 24, the Pharaoh said to his people: "I am your greatest Lord". Allah is simply repeating what the Pharaoh said to his people. Does this mean that Allah agrees that the Pharaoh is the greatest Lord? Definitely not.

After this conversation with this maulvi sahib, I heard a few more times people saying that women are evil because it says in the Quran.

This is the problem with many Muslims. They simply believe what is told to them without going into details or questioning the speaker. In the Muslim culture of the Indian subcontinent, questioning somebody 'higher' than you was/ is regarded as disrespect to him. In my childhood I have heard this shouting, many times:

"Don't interfere when your elders are speaking."

In my practice as a doctor, '*Attention to detail*' was an important ingredient in my approach to the patients' care. I have adopted this attitude when I am studying the Quran and in the important matters of life.

Finally, women are respectable creations of Allah. Whoever looks down on women as 'low' are actually regarding Allah's creation as 'low'. The Quran speaks very highly about "Mariyam" (Mary), mother of Jesus (PBUH) and of "Asiya", the wife of the Pharaoh (66: 11-12). There is a separate chapter named after "Mariyam" (Mary), chapter 19. In addition, Moses' (PBUH) encounter with the girls at the well depicts the decent character of Moses and those girls (28: 22-28).

However, it is also true that in Islam and in other religions, some rules/ regulations are different for women. This is for their safety and because their anatomy, physiology, endocrinology (hormones) and psychology are different from men, also because of how a 'Man' looks at a 'Woman'.

20). Ventilators (Breathing Machines).

Breathing machines are connected to the patient's windpipes in the operation theatres and in the ICU. (Intensive Care Units). They are used if a patient is not breathing sufficiently or is artificially paralysed (artificially induced total body paralysis for major operations) or if the patient is unconscious with impaired breathing, or if the patient is in a coma.

In 2020/21, Covid patients with abnormal blood gases are ventilated till they recover.

There have been some strange encounters with these machines. Some are mine and some are others. Below are a given few:

I). **First time in my life.** In 1973, I was a junior doctor in the Harrogate General Hospital in Yorkshire.

A fifteen-year-old girl was brought to the Accident and Emergency department, unconscious and with very much impaired breathing.

She was the only child of the parents. She went to the dentist to have her tooth removed. The dentist gave her an overdose of the sleeping drug (Barbiturates) and she never woke up.

She was kept in our ICU, ventilated for few days. She never woke up. The consultants did the tests for 'Brain Stem death' and decided to switch off the breathing machine. He filled the legal documents and casually told me: "Azhar, can you switch off the ventilator please" and went off.

I was scared to death. I had never done this before. For the first time in my life, I was going to turn the ventilator off and watch someone dying. I had to do it. I switched off the ventilator. I stood next to her bed, watched her E.C.G. (Heart monitor), and pulse which were getting slower and slower and then they stopped. I stood there for some time, next to her body. As it is, it is difficult to see a dead person, it is much more difficult to see a dying person (since then, I have seen many more). Her parents came in. I admired them so much. They were very calm (unlike what I have seen in India when someone dies). A man was comforting his wife, although she was very quiet as well. Losing your one and only child is not something everyone can bear.

****

Now (2021), when I am writing this, it reminds me of the Prophet of Islam (PBUH) who lost all his children, except one, Fatima (R.A.), during his lifetime. It takes absolute guts to face such things and then carry on with your mission without being ungrateful to God.

One of my friends' fathers lost his son-in-law who was 30 years old. Seeing the pain in the eyes of his daughter, of being a young widow, and knowing that she would never remarry (not allowed in the religion), he stopped believing in God.

Whenever I hear or see on the TV any misfortune or calamity on the individual or on a group of people, like the Fire in Grenfell Tower, Hurricane Harvey and Irma in the Carrabin Islands and the southern United States of America, or the Muslim refugees in Myanmar (Burma), all of these in 2017, I recite various prayers from the Quran which say: *"Allah does not burden any soul more than what it can bear. Oh, our Lord, do not condemn us with misfortunes and calamities which had been on others before us. Do not give us burdens which we cannot bear. Give us strength and patience to stand firm and face boldly any misfortunes and calamities which come to us and not to lose hope in You."*

There are many more prayers like these in the Quran.

II). **All night long.** In my more than 40 years of working life in the operation theatres and in I.C.Us, there have been many occasions when I was up all night, sorting out emergencies, relieving pain in women in labour, delivering babies, retrieving organs, transferring patients to different hospitals, resuscitating patients from the age of neonates to 102 years old, ICU. issues and staff shortage issues (when the night on-call doctor did not turn up).

However, only twice I had to take up the role of a ventilator.

In the early 1980s, I was working at the Royal London Hospital, White chapel, in East London.

I was on call for the night in the ICU. We had a 6-year-old Bengali boy with crushed ribs on the right side as a result of a road traffic accident.

The boy was connected to a child's ventilator. After finishing my rounds at about 11 p.m., I went to my room, which was about 30 seconds walking distance from the ICU. Ten minutes later, the nurse in charge rang me to come to the ICU. urgently. I went there. She told me that the ventilator for the boy has stopped working and she did not know what was wrong with it. I went to the child's bed and took over his ventilation. I asked the nurse to get me another ventilator. There was none. I asked her to call for the engineer to look at the ventilator. After few phone calls, she told me that the engineer could not come until the next day at 8 a.m. I had no choice but to sit next to the boy and hand ventilate him till the next day, 8 a.m. I did this from 11 p.m. till 8 a.m. I had two 10 minutes breaks.

III). All night long…second time.

In 1984 I was working in Saudi Arabia (King Fahad Hospital, Al-Hufuf, Al-Hassa province). One evening, a six-week-old baby was brought for abdominal surgery. In the hospital's A & E, he had an overdose of a drug and stopped breathing. We connected him to the ventilator, which stopped working around 11 p.m. There was no other ventilator available. The mechanic was not able to come till morning 8 a.m. Therefore, I took up the role of the ventilator from 11 p.m. till 8 a.m. without any break. The baby survived without any complications.

IV). New to the ventilator.

This incident was told to me by my consultant when I was a junior doctor in Scotland.

The basic mechanism of 'a' machine is the same, but the controls may be different in different models. For example, the fundamental principles on which an engine of a car runs are the same, but the gear, clutch, light, wipers, and other controls etc., maybe in different places in different models.

Similarly, all microwaves work on the same principle, but the settings and controls may be different in different models.

The same is true with medical machines.

A doctor went to do a locum night shift. In the theatres, he connected the patient to the ventilator. As he was new to the place, people, and the machines, including the ventilator, he could not work out how the ventilator worked. He struggled, panicked but could not work out the ventilator. Apparently, serious harm came to the patient.

My consultant was trying to tell me **PPPPP**. This means Pre-operative Preparations Prevent Pre-operative and Post-operative Problems.

Later, I slightly modified this very good principle for various aspects of life.

V). Wrong connections.

This was also told to me by one of my consultants.

A patient, who happened to be a doctor as well, was on the operating table. At the end of the operation, the anaesthetist gave her 100% oxygen. The patient became blue, dark blue, and darker blue. She never woke up. She was in the I.C.U for few days and then died.

The ventilator was sent for inspection. It emerged that it was serviced a day before and the engineer connected the wrong pipes to the wrong gases' outlets. So, when the anaesthetist pressed for 100% oxygen, 100% nitrous oxide was given to the patient.

This happened more than 40 years ago. Many changes have been brought since then and today's ventilators are very safe and have many safety mechanisms.

There has been no such incidence since then.

VI). Insect causing havoc.

In 2015, I was working in a London hospital. The patient was on the operating table having a major surgery. Through a tube in his windpipe, he was connected to a ventilator. Halfway through the operation, the ventilator started making some funny noises and then stopped. The patient was not getting any oxygen. As I was the senior-most among the doctors in the theatres, I had to sort out the problem, which I did. I disconnected the patient from the ventilator, and I was the ventilator for him until the new one was brought, which took about twenty minutes.

I told the staff to call the engineer from the EBME (Electronic and Bio-medical Engineering) department to look at the old ventilator.

The engineer came and took the ventilator outside the theatres. I went with him as well. The engineer dismantled the machine and after few minutes he found an insect which was stuck in an oxygen pipe. Somehow, it had gone into the machine and travelling through various pipes, it got stuck in the oxygen pipe, blocking the supply to the patient.

No harm had come to the patient.

Medical accidents are exceedingly rare. Operation theatres/ICUs/HDUs are very safe places. Staff are well trained. Especially after Dr Shipman's incident, many safety mechanisms are in place, which ensures that doctors and other health workers are well trained and the instruments and machines are in order.

21). Relocation.

In the same hospital as above, there have been incidences of theft from the male and female changing rooms. In our coffee room, this became a hot topic. One of the lady workers jokingly said: "*Stealing is simply the relocation of the resources*". We all laughed and did not think much about it.

The management was fed up with these thefts. They decided to catch the thieves. There were two thieves, a male worker and the lady who said that stealing is simply the relocation of resources.

They both were "Relocated" elsewhere.

24). "The greatest horse rider" the world had ever seen.

In 1973, I was working in the Harrogate General Hospital, Yorkshire, England.

I was new in the country and homesick. Therefore, apart from studying for my exams, I took some hobbies. One of them was horse riding. I had never done horse riding in my life. I joined a school of Riding. My instructor was a lady…B.

After taking a few lessons, I thought of myself as "The greatest horse rider" the world had ever seen.

One day, I challenged B for a race. She told me not to challenge her. I did not listen and insisted on a race. We both were out in the fields, which were very hilly.

As the race began, B was out of my sight within seconds. My horse was running in some direction. I had totally lost control over her. Samantha (name of my horse) kept running and I was clinging to her back. I had no idea in which direction she was running. Then there was a sudden and very big jolt. I almost fell out of her back. Samantha was standing at the end of a cliff that was more than 100 feet deep. She saved my life. I did not know my way back to the school. The horses are good. Like cats, dogs, pigeons, and other animals, they know their way to their homes. She took me back to the school. B was already there. She kept laughing. She had every right to laugh at me.

Now, in 2021 when I think back, I feel that Man on a whole, especially at a young age, is very 'proud' of himself. He achieves a little and thinks himself 'Great'. He does not know that there is no end to achievements and no matter what he achieves, he should not be proud of himself.

When Neil Armstrong stepped onto the moon, he said: "One small step for man, one giant leap for mankind." The universe is so vast, no matter how many steps man takes; it will always be a small step for Man.

Every religion teaches its followers to be humble.

23). Mohammed Sayed.

This was news on BBC, red button service, on 29-11-2017.

"Mohammed Sayed was born in the USA but was sent to Pakistan by his parents to grow up in Islamic surroundings."

As a young Muslim growing up in Pakistan, he believed in everything thrown on him, in the name of the religion, i.e., Islam.

"Ten years later, when he returned to the US, he gave up Islam, saying that everything he believed, while he was in Pakistan, he now disbelieved."

Comments:

As I have said many times in this book that in the Asian culture, "you do not question your elders, you do not question your religious leaders either. Everything they say is right. You simply accept it." In my personal life, I have questioned many speakers here in London and was told off by others saying, "How dare you question such a great scholar? He has studied religion for seven years, do you know, or does he know?"

As a child and young adult in India, I was not brave enough to question any speaker, though I did have queries /doubts about what they said.

M. Sayed must have heard many things from the maulvis, in the name of the religion, which later, he realised, were simply untrue, unbelievable, and laughable.

I think M. Sayed made the mistake that he did not study the Quran in depth. While in Pakistan, he believed in/kept quiet for everything he heard in the name of religion. Once out in the USA, in the atmosphere of free-thinking, he realised that most of the things he learnt in the name of religion were unbelievable.

While there are so many great scholars in Islam, blind belief in some 'not so great scholars' can mislead you.

Think for yourself. You are responsible for your actions.

24). Friday, 1 December 2017. In the sermon of the Friday prayer, in a mosque, in London E11, the imam said something which I questioned him and then another imam, but they could not come out with a credible explanation.

The story told in the sermon was as follows:

The imam said: "Hell was getting too hot. So, it asked God to do something about it. God told hell that it could breathe twice a year, once to take a breath in and a second time to breathe out. When hell breaths out, it becomes the "summer" season on earth. When it breaths in, it is winter season on earth."

Then the imam said, "look, it is December, it is cold because hell has taken a breath in."

After the prayers, I asked him three questions: **A).** If hell has taken a breath in, causing winter season on the earth, then why Australia, New Zealand and nearby countries are having summer season? **B).** We all know that the sun is the source of heat on the earth. If hell has taken a breath in, causing winter season on the earth, the sun must be hell. The Quran (Chapter 81, Verse 1) and science both say that one day (roughly after 5 billion years, according to **"Sky by night" by Patrick Moore**), the sun will be destroyed, losing all its light and heat. This means hell will no longer be there, therefore where will all the sinners go?

C). If hell's breath is causing summer and winter seasons on the earth, then who is causing the rainy season? In the Indian subcontinent, there are three distinct seasons, from February to the end of May is the summer season, June to September is the rainy season, and October to the end of January is the winter.

The imam could not answer these three questions. I asked these questions to another imam of another mosque; he could not answer them either.

Here lies the problem. People simply believe in everything they hear in the name of Islam. They are told to believe because everyone around them believes. However, people like Mohammed Sayed, once they are out of their 'surroundings', start disbelieving in everything.

The imams study in religious schools for five to seven years. Out of these three years, they spend memorising the Quran, which is great, a big achievement and service to the community. The knowledge they acquire in the rest of the years is a mixture of facts and not so facts. Only a small portion is true and facts, the rest is a matter of interpretation, therefore could be doubtful, may have an alternative explanation, or maybe totally untrue.

People like Mohamed Sayed probably focus on such doubtful/unbelievable things and then disbelieve in everything, thinking, "Is this Islam?" If they study the Quran and get the fundamentals right, they will disbelieve 'fictions' and have a firm belief in 'facts'.

If I am running a "Madrassah" (Islamic Religious School), I will introduce two subjects, General knowledge and Basic sciences.

25). What a great difference.

In September 1973, I was a surgical house officer in the Kings Lynn general hospital, Norfolk, England. In those days, in this part of the country, there were hardly any Asians.

Once, a patient, an Englishman, was admitted to the ward. My consultant sent me to take the history, examine the patient, write a provisional diagnosis, order investigations, and prescribe the appropriate treatment and then inform the consultant.

I approached the patient. When he saw me, he said: "I do not want to talk to or be touched by a coloured man." I reported this to the consultant, and he sorted out the matter. This was my first encounter with racial abuse/insults.

In the same ward, sometime later, another English gentleman was admitted. He was not my patient. I noticed that he did not have any visitors. Apparently, he had no close relatives. As I came to know that he had a terminal illness and did not have much time in this world, I felt sorry for him and started seeing him and chatting with him in my off time. We became close 'friends'. He was in his 70s, and I was in my 20s. One day I told him that I had finished my job in the hospital and was going to leave soon. He was sad to hear this and said: "I am very lonely; I have no one in this world. I have a fair amount of estate; can I write your name in my will? I want you to inherit it. You have been very kind to me." I was shocked. I said, "no way."

Although I was young and immature and new in England, I knew that in situations like these, after the death of the person, suddenly many 'caring' relatives appear to claim the estate. I have seen this in India.

I left the hospital, praying for him to have a peaceful, pain-free death.

There are good and bad people in every society.

Friday, 27/10/2017 B.B.C. red button world news:

Israel honours a Muslim, Arab, holocaust saviour.

Egyptian doctor Mohammed Helmy saved a Jewish woman and her family in Berlin in the 2nd world war. Some 70 Muslims are among 26,500 non-Jewish people recognised by Israel as saviours.

A descendent of Dr Helmy, who died in 1982, received the award.

Elsewhere, in this book, I have written that in India, during Hindu-Muslim riots, in the 1950s and 60s, there was a gesture of goodwill from both sides. Quite a few Hindus saved Muslims and vice versa.

26). Name and fame:

There is always a bit of luck in everything we get/do not get in life. Name and Fame is not an exception to this.

Psychologically, it is an inner desire of every human being to be 'Famous', 'Known'.

January 2018. A surgeon, Mr Simon Bramhall, in Birmingham's Queen Elizabeth hospital, UK, was taken to court for writing his initials on two patient's livers during a liver transplant operation.

The TV reporter brought some other patients of the same surgeon and interviewed them. They were extremely grateful to the surgeon, speaking in support of him and said, "he saved our lives."

Behind the scenes.

Although Mr Bramhall was the surgeon who transplanted the livers, but what the patients do not know that it is the entire team in the operation theatres which saves patients' lives. The team members do not get any "name and fame."

To start with, in this case, the two people who agreed to donate their livers saved two lives.

In addition to this, every single department in a hospital does a great job in saving patients' lives. This includes haematology, biochemistry, pathology, radiology, pharmacy and many more. They all go unknown. Without their support, no surgery will be successful. They do a great job. With their support only, a greater job is done in the operation theatres.

However, the greatest job is done in the ICU. (Intensive Care Unit). After any major surgery, patients go to the ICU. and it is the work done there which saves the patient's life. Nobody knows them.

Extremely acutely ill patients with minute-by-minute changing pathology/ physiology are treated in the ICU. It is the expertise of the ICU staff which saves lives.

There is 1 to 1 care, 24/7. In the UK, this is all free, thanks to the 'Great NHS'.

This way, the NHS is the greatest public service, free of charge in the UK. In many other countries, this treatment is extremely expensive. Even in the UK, only the NHS has this kind of facility. The private sector (private hospitals), which I came in contact with, depend on the NHS hospitals when things go wrong. I know quite a few patients who were transferred from private hospitals to NHS hospitals when they needed ICU treatment.

(The NHS is the third-largest public sector employer in the world, with the Chinese army being the first and the Indian Railways being the second).

Coming back to name and fame, once I had a patient, in London, an English man, a civil engineer, who came for surgery.

Talking to me in the operation theatres, he appreciated and admired what a great job 'Doctors' do, especially those in the operation theatres. Then he started feeling guilty as to why he was not a doctor; he could have done a great job.

I told him: "Look around, see this wonderful building of hospital and operation theatres; if there are no civil engineers, who design and build all this, we, the doctors, won't be able to do any work. Look at the instruments, if there are no mechanical engineers and factory workers, we cannot do anything. Look at the monitors in the operation theatres, if there are no electrical and electronic engineers, we cannot do anything. Look at all the drugs we use. If there are no scientists and pharmaceutical companies, we cannot do anything. The place is clean, if there are no cleaners, we cannot do anything. The porters bring and take the patients to the wards. Without them, no patient would be in the operation theatre." The fact is that in the world, everyone who works is important, even though he may not be known.

God, in His wisdom, has distributed work among people and name and fame.

The patient was very grateful to me and said not many doctors take time to talk to patients like this. His surgery was successful, and he went home safe and sound and feeling happy that he was important in society, although unknown.

The heads of states, secretaries of states and ministers are famous and known in the world. However, they cannot do anything if there are no civil servants, who are totally unknown.

There is always a bit of luck in this world, what you get and do not get. Fame is not an exception to this; however, worldly fame has no value in the eyes of God.

What God values, who is more honest, sincere, and pious: Surah 49, verse 13.

27) Minister for the lonely.

Front page of the Daily Mail, British newspaper, Wednesday, 17-01-2018. The UK government has appointed a minister, Tracey Crouch, to tackle the problem of loneliness and social isolation, which is affecting nine million adults in Britain.

According to Age UK, 200,000 older people have not had a conversation with a relative or friend for more than a month.

This is not a new problem.

I have seen loneliness in old people in India. They suffer in silence, as this is not regarded as a problem, the attitude was: "What can anyone do? Everyone is busy, they (old people) have to somehow tolerate it."

In the late 1970s, I was working in the A & E in Medway, Gillingham, Kent. At 3 a.m., a young girl was brought to A & E. She called the ambulance as she was getting panicky. I talked to her, and she said that she was very lonely and just wanted to talk to someone.

"Loneliness is killing everyone" is a famous song in a Bollywood movie called Red. The song is in Hindi/Urdu, but the title wordings are in English. The heroine gets into the wrong hands and becomes an alcoholic because of loneliness.

Some time ago, I read in a magazine that in northern European countries, the suicide rate increases in the winter months as a result of loneliness and long, cold nights.

My son is a GP, and he says that these days, for older people, we look for: physical health, mental health, and social health. The word social health was new to me. When I was studying medicine in India (1960s), there was no concept of 'social health'. My son explained to me how social isolation can lead to mental health problems.

Factors limiting socialisation.

In my view, socialisation is limited by various factors. The most important one is 'culture' and not religion nor language.

I am Asian, from India. My neighbours are non-Asians. Although I have been living next to them for the last 35 years, there is only Hello and Hi, or a short chat with them, if met them on the road. However, I travel 20+ miles to see friends who are of Indian origin. They are not all Muslims. My son has a Hindu friend in Manchester. His mother died back in Mauritius. My son travelled from London to Manchester to offer his condolences.

My next-door neighbour died. As our terms were only Hello and Hi, we were not invited to the funeral. The phrase: "Birds of the same feathers flock together" is very true, but it can be a barrier in socialisation and therefore creates loneliness.

The problem with differing cultures is, there is always a sense of unease or scepticism. If you are more open about your cultural/religious beliefs, this may help in mixing with people of different cultures. Sensible, educated people will accept it and respect it.

When my daughter got married, I invited my English colleagues from the hospital and told them that in our culture, men and women do not shake hands or dance together. They respected it. However, this is not always the case. I used to call them for dinner at home. I stopped it because some of them commented, "the food was very nice, but there was no alcohol."

There is a 'good' human being inside every person. This is because; Man was created with the best of the moulds (surah 95, verse 4). It is the surroundings and upbringing which create 'dents' in the mould. These dents are prejudice against race, gender, religion, colour, culture, superiority complex, jealousy, greed, competition with each other, etc. If one can mend (fight) these dents, he will come out as the original 'good' human being. This is a test for human beings on earth. There are so many examples of this:

On Leytonstone high road, London E11, there is a mosque. I go there with my family for Friday prayers. An Asian Muslim person who is wheelchair-bound is brought to the mosque by a Christian fellow who stays there in the mosque till the prayers are finished.

I was in Hyderabad, India on an Eid occasion. The place for the Eid prayer was full of Muslims, in their thousands, and in between the rows and surrounding them were the Hindu police officials, with rifles, guarding them. In a Hindu country, Hindus are guarding the Muslims so that they can pray in peace.

I saw a documentary in which the Sikhs from India go to Pakistan to visit their sacred places and they are guarded by Muslim Pakistani police. There are good people everywhere because the origin of man was good. There is no fault in God's creation, Surah 67, verse 3.

Coming back to the loneliness and isolation, whatever the government plans to do is a good and a positive step. However, can every individual do something about it? Yes.

If you are an atheist, you can still help older people in your community, based on humanity, feeling for them and by remembering that one day you will be old.

For those who believe in God, look into your religious book. Every religion teaches you to be social, help the old and vulnerable people, especially your parents.

In Surah 31, verses 12-19, Luqman (A.S.) is advising his son. Among various advice, he says, verse 18: *Do not turn your face away from people.*"

In Surah 17, Verse 23 and 24, Allah says:

"And your Lord has decreed that you worship none but Him and be dutiful to your parents. If one or both of them reach old age, respect them, not shout at them and address them in terms of honour. Lower yourself in front of them with humility and say…Oh my Lord, have mercy on them as they had mercy on me when bringing me up."

In the 2nd Surah, verse 27, it is said: "…and those who sever the relations which Allah has ordained to keep…they are the losers.

In a Hadith, the Prophet (PBUH) said: "After the death of your parents, there are three things you can do to comfort their souls. One of these is to keep good terms and help their relatives and friends."

Almost certainly, the relatives and friends of anyone's parents are of the same age as the parents, and as old as the parents were. This way, old people will have someone to take care of them and talk to them.

I am sure this sort of teaching is there in other religious scriptures as well.

1-02-2018. BBC News: A survey done by the mental health campaign, "Time to change", found that 2/3 of the adults in Britain have no one to talk to about their problems. The reasons are busy life and other commitments.

10 October 2018. Prime minister **Theresa May** appointed Jackie Doyle Price as "Minister for prevention of suicide" on world mental health day.

Will it work? To some extent…yes. It is a good step, but more steps are to be taken by immediate family and friends.

28). British values:

1-02-2018. BBC News, channel 130, at 8:15 pm.

"Religious extremists are targeting schools to undermine the British values."

This was the only sentence read by the newscaster.

My comments:

The questions which came to my mind were:

1. What is the definition of values?
2. What is the definition of "British Values?"
3. Who determines these values?
4. How are they determined?

5. When were they determined?
6. What happened if the British values clash with the religious beliefs or the culture? What do you follow?
7. Where is the freedom to practice your beliefs and culture?
8. What happens if someone, a British citizen, does not follow these values?
9. Does the Magna Carta protect individuals from following these values?
10. Values change with time. Do we have to follow the values drawn some time ago? Britain today is a multi-faith, multi-ethnic and multi-cultural society.

I do not know the answers, nor did the BBC explain them in its news.

29). A Few days to live, admiration, and the lessons:
02-02-2018. BBC News headlines.

Deaths by prostate cancer have exceeded the deaths by breast cancer. This was the headline. This was followed by a discussion and interview with the patients.

One patient, a young Englishman, was interviewed. I was deeply moved and impressed by him and admire his courage. He was diagnosed with this cancer and was too late to have any curative treatment. He had limited time in this world. He was shown jogging in a park, like any other jogger.

During the interview, he was very calm, quiet, and collected. He was smiling and chatting normally, advising other patients. Most will go into panic or extreme depression.

5 September 2018. BBC News headlines.

Rachael Bland, the BBC Radio 5 live presenter, has died this morning of breast cancer, aged 40.

I have been following her story ever since she was told that she had few days to live. What a brave and courageous lady. She took death so bravely and calmly and prepared for her son, Freddie, whatever she could. She called D-day, Death Day. It takes a lot to do this. Freddie will grow without her but will always be proud of his brave mother.

As a doctor, in my years of hospital work, I have seen many people dying. The reaction of their relatives was quite different. In general, people in the West take death as a natural phenomenon and accept it, do not show any overwhelming emotions. However, in the East, the reaction is very different and quite the opposite to that of the West.

What is the reason? Closed family? Cultural impact? Religious teachings and fear of how the deceased would be treated in the hereafter?

Probably a psychologist will be able to explain better.

30). Sharia courts in Britain.

The latest news, on 2/2/2018, is that the UK government rejects calls to legitimise sharia courts in Britain. I am not surprised, and I am not unhappy either.

People who run sharia courts and act as the judges, giving Fatwas are, in many cases, not well versed in either Islamic law nor British law. Their fatwas are based on which school of thought they belong to. The majority of Asians belong to the Hanafi School of Thought and non-Asians are either Shafa'e, or Malaki, or Humbali. They all have their own laws and give fatwas according to the teachings of their school. To this are added personal views of the person giving fatwa. Their fatwas are very strict with no consideration to the current situation and no flexibility.

Example: 1. A person was strongly against Muslims watching TV. He used to stay at the exit of the mosque and used to say to everyone going out after prayers: "Watching TV is haram, watching TV is haram."

One day he told me that if he had power, he would take a bulldozer and demolish all the Muslim houses which have TV. This is his sharia law.

Example: 2. At the end of the mid-day prayer, the imam announced that everyone should sign the petition near the exit door. This was about not to agree to have a post-mortem done on deceased Muslims. This is his sharia law.

Example: 3. According to British law, when a man dies, all his assets go to his wife. When she dies, then the assets are distributed as per will. However,

Hanafi School Sharia law says that the assets of a deceased person should be distributed as soon as possible after his death. This can cause problems.

Example:

Person "A" has an asset of £ 400,000 in the form of the house in which he has been living with his wife. He has three children. They live separately, in their own homes. "A" dies, leaving behind a wife and three children. If the assets have to be distributed soon after his death, the house needs to be sold. The house is sold for £ 400,000. The wife will get £ 50,000, as per Sharia law, rest is distributed among children. Now the wife has no house to live in, has only £ 50,000 to live for the rest of her life. She cannot buy even a room in £ 50,000. What is she going to do? Beg one of the children to keep her in his house? This is cruel and impractical. A sharia court will give this decision, with no consideration to the wife and her problems.

The solution would be that the wife stays in her husband's house until her death and then the assets will be distributed.

When I discussed this scenario with an imam of Hanafi School, his answer was: "the wife, somehow, will have to survive, but the assets must be distributed soon after A's death." Here again, there is no consideration and sympathy to a woman.

Example: 4. Divorce. The ruling by the Supreme Court in India in late 2017 is a landmark and a victory for the truth.

The imams I talked to here in London are very unhappy with this ruling and will still give a fatwa based on their version of sharia law, i.e., three divorces from 'man', in one go is the final divorce, even though it is against the Quran.

You go to any sharia court; the majority of complaints are from women against their husbands or brothers or fathers.

Example: 5. Inheritance to grandchildren. The opinion is divided with strict Hanafi muftis saying that grandchildren have no rights, except what a man wants to give from his 1/3 portion. I believe the Egyptians have modified this ruling.

The truth is that these four schools of thought evolved centuries ago, in the Middle East, taking into consideration the circumstances and needs at that time. They do not have credible answers to all the problems we have in the 21st century.

My prediction is that with time, these schools will fade away and new schools will evolve.

I am a practising Muslim, and I am happy that the government decided not to legitimise/recognise sharia courts.

31). Export, import:

February 2018 news. Australia, within ten years, will be among the top ten countries which export arms.

My only comment is: "And Muslim countries will be among top 50 countries which will import these arms so that they can kill each other."

32). Muslim scientists…what went wrong?

Recently, in February 2018, I read a book in Urdu named "Muslim scientists", written by Sayyed Mujibuddin, published by Facts publications, Temple Road, Lahore, Pakistan.

In this book, the writer wrote about the great Muslim scientists and their achievements. It is a very good book and shows the bright 'past' of Muslims.

These scientists achieved many milestones in various branches of science like Physics, Chemistry, Maths, Geometry, Algebra, Medicine and much more.

These scientists were good, practising Muslims as well, who understood Islam very well and knew the Fiqh (rules, regulations, laws, halal, haram etc.) very well. The ruler, governors and other well-off people of their times encouraged them and helped them in any way they could.

When I read all of this, the question which came to my mind was: "What went wrong? Why, in today's world, are there hardly any Muslim scientist's names? Who is responsible for this?"

God has given our religious leaders a very special place in the community. They have the privilege of addressing hundreds of people, not just once or twice but fifty-two times a year, i.e., every Friday, and many times in Ramadhan and on many other occasions like Eid days. What they say is subconsciously absorbed by the people.

While they say many good things, which we have heard hundreds of times, they never mention the importance of worldly education, especially science and technology. Most of them are against this education. They do not understand the importance of these subjects because of what they learn in their Madrassahs.

Once, I said to an imam that there are so many scientific programmes available on TV like Horizon, Equinox, tomorrow's world, trust me, I am a doctor, discovery channels and many more. Those who do not know much about science should take advantage of these programmes.

On the following Friday, in his speech (sermon of Friday prayer), he said, addressing to an audience of about four hundred people, that we have nothing to do with science, we do not have to know the life cycle of mice, we have come in this world only to keep saying Allah, Allah. Such messages, subconsciously, affects people's minds. No wonder why Muslims are right at the back of the queue when it comes to science and technology.

Sometime ago, there was a survey done in England which showed that Asian children are doing very well in schools. Going into details, these children were mainly of Chinese and Indian origin. It was specifically said that they were not of Pakistani nor Bangladeshi origin. No wonder why India has come up as the world's top three developing industrial nation.

From my childhood in India, 1954 till now in 2018, in England, I have felt that Muslim religious leaders are very suspicious of 'western education'. Learning the English language was declared as a sin, English being the language of infidels. They think that western education destroys the Muslim faith and Muslim values. In support of their arguments, they say that western education believes in Darwin's theory of evolution, it promotes sex education in schools, encourages mixed gatherings etc.

To this, I say that no man is perfect, no nation is perfect. There is good and not so good in everyone. You take what is good in others and leave what you think is bad. By keeping away from western education, you are missing out on many good things they can offer.

I have been to many science museums, in Hyderabad, in London, and in other places.

Mufti Taqi Usmani, in his book "Jahn-e-deedah" (one who has seen the whole world) on page 586 onwards, writes about the science centre in Toronto, Canada. It is a four-story building full of scientific discoveries and inventions.

However, one noticeable thing in these museums is that none of the discoveries and inventions was made by Muslims.

Muslims had a glorious past, thanks to those scientists. Without science, they have a bleak future.

Recently, I read two more books about Muslim scientists. One is "The famous Muslim scientists" by the same author as the first book, "Great Muslim scientists" and the second one is, "1001 Inventions. Muslim Heritage in our world." 2nd edition. The chief editor is Saleem T.S. Al Hassani, issued by the Foundation of Science, Technology and civilisation.

Altogether, the three books which I read on the topic of 'Muslim scientists' consists of about 1000 pages. I can summarise these 1000 pages in one sentence:

"Once upon a time, Muslims were great."

The same theme is written by Allama Iqbal, the poet of the east.
"They were your forefathers, who are you, what are you?"

32). Why I left the preaching party.

The preaching party is made up of a group of Asian Muslims, who go round preaching Islam to Muslims only. I joined this party in the 1960s in Hyderabad, India, when I was doing my 'O' levels. They have a book which they believe to be true word for word. In the mosques which allow them to have their activities (not all mosques allow them), they have their gatherings after the obligatory prayers in which the same speech is repeated again and again. Then they go out in groups of three or more to various houses of Muslims (only) to preach Islam. In the group of three, one person is the leader, the second one is the guide and the third one is the speaker.

In India, I had done this many times.

Here in the UK I had been to Bolton, Bury, and Blackburn and nearby places on a 'preaching tour'. As an immature, inexperienced 'O' level student in India, I believed everything they said and everything written in their book. In Indian culture in those days and probably even now, you are not allowed to disagree with adults.

However, as my life progressed, I qualified as a doctor, came to the UK, did further studies, i.e., Fellow of the Faculty of Anaesthetics of the Royal College of Surgeons; (F.F.A.R.C.S) in my field and started thinking seriously about this party. Then I left the party. The reasons were:

1. They preach Islam to Muslims only. This is surprising, but they say that those Muslims who have forgotten their religion and are Muslims by name only are the target.

My family and I go to the mosque regularly and follow Islamic principles in practical life. Yet the people from this preaching party come to my house as well to preach me, Islam. I asked them why they come to preach to me when I am already practising Islam. The answer I got was: "...but you are not practising the correct Islam, and this is what we want to teach you."

This was very annoying. They say that unless you follow the correct Islam, and ours is the correct Islam only, you are doomed. I had a big 'go' at them and told them about the many flaws in their practice of Islam.

1. Whenever they came to my house, I asked them that my neighbours are non-Muslims, why did they not preach Islam to them? The answer was: "We want to correct you first." They have been correcting me for the last thirty-odd years without success. The fact is:

2. Their knowledge of Islam is very poor. They cannot come up with decent, logical, well-articulated arguments in favour of Islam.

3. Their emphasis is on appearance and rituals only. In the name of the Sunnah (way of Prophet's life), they say things which I disagree with and many others too.

4. Their knowledge of the Quran is very poor too. In their preaching, they do not come out with any verses of the Quran. In fact, quite a few members of the party cannot read the Quran properly.

5. All their points are from a book; written by two Indian 'scholars'. I can find so many flaws in that book. I told them that this book was written by human beings, so it has defects and mistakes in it; it should not be taken word for word to be true. The reply was: "But they are great scholars; how can they be wrong?" They do not want to hear anything against the book or its author.

7. See chapter 18, page 110, "My GP friend." He was a continually active member of this party. He believed in every single word of the book of this party and every single word which came out from the *Ameer* (leader) of the party.

8. The party members and their teachings distract the students from their studies. They brain-wash to say that this world is not worth living, so do not do any work for it. All your work should be for the hereafter. Their slogan is: "*Work for this world, for as much as you live here, work for the Aakhira (hereafter) for as much as you live there.*"

In Hyderabad, under the influence of this party, some university students left their studies completely. The parents were cursing the party.

9. They neglect their families and their needs. They go away on a long preaching tour (40 days), leaving wives and children at home. Wives need husbands, and children need fathers.

10. A 'feel-good factor' is created in the atmosphere of their gathering. People feel compelled to say yes to everything said in the gathering. People feel happy that "Oh, yes, we are doing something for Islam."

11. I know quite a few converted (reverted) Muslims, and I also read a book by Dr Abdul Ghani Farooq, *Why we converted to Islam*". None of these newly converted Muslims accepted Islam as a result of the efforts of this preaching party. They do not preach to non-Muslims.

12. I also saw few programmes on TV about the Muslims who left Islam. Where was the preaching party?

13. The most annoying for me when I was a member of this party was that they, the senior members, did not allow me to ask questions or raise concerns or challenge their teachings.

14. I never ever heard a single word from the speakers of this party about the importance of "worldly education", especially the sciences and technology. I heard the contrary statements that science and technology is nothing to do with us. It is the job for non-Muslims. This concept is 100% un-Islamic.

15. Once, the party members came to my house and the 'speaker' said, "I have come from the frontier, Pakistan, all the way to London, to teach you, Islam." Then he said the fundamentals of Islam, which I already knew. I asked him: "Who is looking after your wife and children? Providing daily bread." The answer was "Allah". I asked him how he funded his journey. He said that he had a piece of land, which he sold.

To me, his understanding of Islam was very poor, very distorted, without common sense.

16. A member of this party left his wife and children here in the UK and went on a preaching tour to Bangladesh for six months. He came back with T.B. and died soon after.

Saying all this about the party, I found that the members are innocent and honest people who do not think much.

A cricketer and a film actress, who were born Muslims but not practising, came back to practising Islam because of the efforts of this party. These are the only two positive results I heard about.

Overall, the party is not for me. It is not for those who think, it is for those who simply follow.

33). Medications in Ramadhan.

I worked in the Newham teaching hospital, London E13 8SL, for 27 years. Every year, before the month of Ramadhan, a special presentation is given in the Grand Rounds regarding Ramadhan and how to adjust medications during fasting and any related issues. I have not seen this in India when I was doing my basic medical degree and training there. I have not heard of this in any Muslim country either.

The **BMA** (British Medical Association) also holds such presentations. There is one on 18-04-2018.

This country, the UK, looks after its citizens very well regardless of their origin, beliefs, ethnicity etc. Muslims must be grateful for this service.

Adjusting medications during Ramadhan is an important issue, especially for diabetics, those with heart conditions, and kidney problems.

Please talk to your GP if you have any concerns regarding your medications and fasting.

34). You must know me…(desire for name and fame).

Here in London, I was sitting with a friend in his house, who is a lawyer. Another man came to his house. My lawyer friend introduced me to him, saying, "This is Mr So and so." After the greetings, the man told me: "You must know me." I told him that sorry, but I did not know him. He said quite aggressively: "No, it is not possible that you don't know me." I told him again that I did not know him. His face got puffed up, and he looked very angry. After a few moments of silence, he said: "Don't you know me? I am the ex-announcer of Radio Pakistan."

I could not believe the way he behaved.

Because of my Muslim name, he straight away assumed that I am from Pakistan.

Did he not know that India still has a large population of Muslims?

Being a Muslim, did he not know that the Quran, in many places, teaches not to be proud of what you are, your position, your wealth etc.? This is the teaching of all religions.

Did he not see around, in the world, that many famous faces have come and gone? Nobody remembers them. What is an announcer? What is his value when Kings are buried under tonnes of mud? Nobody remembers them...who cares?

I have come across quite a few people like this, unfortunately, mostly Muslims. This is human nature; psychology...desire to be known and famous...have authority over others.

One of the consultant surgeons, a non-Muslim in the North of England, was very proud of his position and what he could do as a surgeon. He treated everyone as 'dirt'. He used to call himself 'God'. Once, an unusually difficult case was on the operation table. The 'God' was shivering like anything. We thought he was going to wet himself or was going to have a heart attack.

"Do not walk on the face of the earth with pride..." Surah 31, verse 18, 19.

"What is with you in this world will perish, what you leave with God will last." Surah 16, verse 96.

See also chapter 8, page 76: "You don't know who I am."

35). You are not good enough.

Near my house in London, a non-Muslim boy fell in love with a Muslim girl.

The girl was also in love with him. When it came to marriage, the girl insisted that he converts to Islam.

In love, especially of teenage, the man, and probably woman, can do anything and agrees to any terms and conditions.

The boy converted to Islam, started going to the mosque and started learning about Islam. Then he told the girl that she was not a "good enough Muslim, she would have to change, otherwise, he won't marry her." The girl did not agree, and he left her; he married some other Muslim girl.

36). Bacon, sausages and alcohol.

News on 26-05-2018 (I read this news on my desktop)

"No amount of bacon, sausages and alcohol is safe to consume." These are the new guidelines from the World Cancer Research Fund.

In Islam, all of these are prohibited.

A car manufacturer knows more about the car and its engine, how to handle it and how to maintain it. What to do and what not to do. The person who drives the car does not have this knowledge. The only way he can keep the car up to date is to follow the instructions given by the manufacture in the manual.

Similarly, God created us. He knows more about our body and soul than we know. The only way our body and soul will run smoothly when we follow the instructions from the manufacturer, i.e., God, in His manual. For Muslims, the manual is the holy Quran.

To get the full benefits, you need to follow the manual completely. This is mentioned in Surah 2, verse 208, *"Oh, you believers, enter into Islam completely..."*, meaning follow the entire manual, not just the bits and pieces which are easy or which you like, or which suits you.

If a non-Muslim follows the principles, i.e., does not drink alcohol, does not gamble etc., he will get all the benefits. This is because what is given in the manual can be called 'laws of nature', which are there for everyone, not just for Muslims.

37). What a contrast.

May 2018 (Ramadhan 1439 AH).

I was watching a series of programmes on BBC, I-Player about "Astronauts, do you have what it takes to be?", a very interesting and educational series. It showed how astronauts are selected to go to the ISS (International Space Station).

Then I watched a series of programmes on YouTube. It was about Pakistani so-called religious scholars criticising, condemning each other and throwing filth on each other on various religious issues.

The West has advanced because the West does not fight on religious issues and it knows the importance of science and technology.

Muslim countries are right at the back in everything in the world because they fight on religious issues and have not yet understood the importance of science and technology.

38). Slave's mind (five stories)

a) Asian senior, English junior

In a London hospital, I was on call for the weekend, and I had an English/white junior doctor working with me.

While seeing patients, I told an Asian patient's relatives that the patient was not progressing very well, and we needed to shift him to a tertiary centre. The relatives were not happy, and they complained to the manager, who was an English man as well and knew me very well.

The manager came to me. We had very friendly relations. He told me not to worry. "I know how to sort this out." He said, "I will send your junior, the English junior doctor, to tell them that the patient needs to be shifted to a teaching hospital. They will agree. I know these people. They were not happy with non-white nurses looking after their patients either. They want an 'All white' team."

The junior went and told them that the patient needed to be shifted to a teaching hospital. Happily, the relatives agreed (a white doctor told us; he cannot be wrong). Guess what was the religion of the patient and his relatives? ...Yes, your guess is right. They were Muslims from a country in the Indian subcontinent.

b) During my annual leave, I went back to Hyderabad, India, to see my parents and sisters.

During an evening gathering with other relatives and friends, they asked me about my work in the UK. I told them that I work in the operation theatres, ICU, resuscitation rooms and labour ward (at that time, I was a junior doctor).

One of the friends looked very uncomfortable and was making faces. I asked him what the matter was.

He said, "How can you work in such an acute, delicate, life and death speciality?"

I asked him, "Why not?"

His answer was, "Oh, you need to be highly qualified to work in this speciality. It is for white people only."

c) As a junior doctor, I was preparing for my fellowship examination. One of my close relatives, whom I always thought was my well-wisher, kept discouraging me. His standard sentences were, "Why are you studying? You won't pass; only intelligent people pass; only white people pass the FRCS examination."

This he repeated many times. While I was studying in my room, he would come, stand at the door, and repeat these sentences. This was his daily routine till I moved out of his house. Not only this reflects a slave's mind, but it also reflects the jealously in human nature (This 'built-in' feature of human nature can be and should be overcome with active efforts).

Here is a joke:

A man died and was taken up by the angels. He asked angels to see hell, so he was taken for a tour of hell.

"This place, a deep well, is for non-Muslims", the angels said. There were many other angels guarding the place. "What are they for?" asked the man.

"So that no one would escape," the angels said.

Then he was taken to another well. "This well is for those who did not believe in God," the angels said. Here again, angels were guarding the well so that no-one would escape.

Lastly, the man was taken to a well. "This is for Muslims", the angels said. There were no angels guarding the well. The man asked why? Angels told him, "Look down the well, you will know."

The man looked down. He saw that whenever a Muslim was trying to climb up the well to escape, ten Muslims were pulling him down.

This is jealousy; they cannot see anyone better off than themselves.

d). Onion and white man.

In Hyderabad, one lady was cutting the onions to make curry. Tears were coming from her eyes, the reaction was due to the onions' vapours.

I told her that it should be possible to make a device that would solve the problem of the vapour going into the eyes. Her answer reflected the typical Asian Muslim mentality. She said, "Such a device will be invented when a white man starts using onions at a large scale."

e) In chapter 3, page 58 (Scholar from South Africa), I have written that I was invited to attend a talk by this 'scholar' in the mosque with the wordings: "Doctor Sahib, the speaker is very knowledgeable, he speaks in English."

Are 70 years of independence not enough to get rid of a slave's mind?

What I find quite funny is that in the mosques, non-Muslims are condemned for being non-Muslims. Yet, at the announcement time, the imam says that so and so, our Muslim brother/sister is very ill, having a major operation, is in the ICU, etc., do pray for his/her health, for the speedy recovery etc. What the imam does not know that majority of the health professionals looking after these very ill Muslim patients in the operation theatre and ICU are non-Muslims, who have been condemned a minute ago.

39. Coronavirus…A conspiracy against Muslims?

August 2020. This is what I have heard from some (not all) worshipers and an imam:

Imam: "Coronavirus is nothing but a conspiracy against Muslims."

I: "How? And do you have any proof?"

Imam: "They (government) has banned congregational prayers. Only Muslims do congregational prayers."

I: "Christians do on Sundays, that is banned as well."

Imam: "They have closed mosques, banned shaking hands, banned standing shoulder to shoulder during prayers (in the name of social distancing). These are all Sunnah (Prophetic way of life) and "they, the government," are bringing all these rules, in the name of Coronavirus, to destroy Islam, our way of life."

I: "But pubs are closed, social distancing is for everyone, shops are closed, essential shops have strict rules, and these rules are for everyone. How are they going to destroy Islam and the Muslim way of life by closing pubs? How many Muslims go to the pubs?"

Imam: "You don't know, they are very clever, they know everything about us."

I: "They, 'the Government', has brought furlough scheme, Muslims are using this scheme as well, to get by with their daily needs. Chancellor of the exchequer, Rishi Sunak has rolled out the "Eat out to help out" scheme where you get a 50% discount on your meals. Muslims are benefiting from this scheme as well. How is all this going to destroy Islam and Muslims? How kind is this enemy of Islam (government) that it is feeding you while you sit at home, taking care of you when you are ill. What kind of conspiracy against Muslims is this? That even non-Muslims are dying as well?"

No answer. After a while, the Imam said: "Scientists say there is going to be another wave of Coronavirus in December."

I: "You mean 'they' are going to bring another conspiracy against Muslims in December, and they are so stupid that they are telling Muslims well beforehand that this is going to happen in December. Does this make any sense?"

The imam kept quiet. After a while, he agreed that what I said made sense and apologised. I appreciated this act from this imam. He understood that his theory of conspiracy was wrong. Other worshipers did not agree with me and still think "they, the government" are out to destroy Islam and Muslims and the Coronavirus is nothing but a hoax. They said to me, "You don't understand 'them', doctor sahib, they are very deep." I asked for proof, and they had none.

I respect our imams because a) they are pious people; their piety is above average. b) They are Hafiz (memorised the whole Quran in order, word for word) which is a big achievement. My respect ends here. What they say in their sermons or privately is a mixture of truth and not so truth or silly. They need to understand the importance of science and know what is going on in the world and improve their general knowledge. They need to take advantage of the facilities available and improve their general knowledge and, in fact, their understanding of Islam. When Tim Peak, the British astronaut, went to the ISS (International Space Station), I mentioned this in the mosque and the reaction was, "It is nothing to do with us."

To be fair, not all imams are like what I have mentioned above. Few do have a good understanding of what is going on around them and what is needed to be done.

Chapter Twenty
Fact or Fiction?

Scholars or storytellers? Made-up miracles?

18 strange but not true stories.

I read a variety of books that come under the common heading of 'Islamic literature'. I listen to many imams and speakers who come under the group of 'Islamic scholars'. I sit in the Islamic gatherings in which books written by so-called 'scholars' are read without questioning.

While most books and speakers are good and sensible, others are not.

Going through some of the so-called 'Islamic literature' and listening to some of the so-called 'Islamic scholars', I find it difficult to believe some (not all) of the things they write and speak. Some I have already written in other chapters like MRI and tiger, Jins did it, Scholars from India and South Africa, Professor of physics and 666, etc.

It is not possible for me to give references to all the stories I am writing below. I read the books and heard from speakers over a period of 30 years or more. However, they are all either from what I have read or heard from speakers.

In my view, they are all fiction. However, in the authors/speakers' views, they are all facts. I leave the readers to decide.

Here are some of the stories:

a. All problems, one solution.

This was a Friday prayer's sermon in a London E11 mosque. The Imam started saying how bad the state of Muslims in today's world was. We (Muslims) are uneducated, unemployed, weak, suppressed by everyone. We have no voice, no value, and no power. We have many social problems at home; our youngsters have lost their ways and are worthless. Parents did not guide their children because they themselves were lost.

190

He went on and on about the 'bad' situation in which Muslims were in the world. Then he said, "There is one and only one reason for this and there is one and only one solution to this." Then there was a long pause.

I was convinced that he was going to say that the one and only reason for all the problems with Muslims was, 'They have forgotten the Quran'. I was absolutely sure that he would quote this verse from Surah 25, verse 30, in which the Prophet (PBUH) would complain to Allah, on the day of judgement, saying, *"Oh My Lord, these are my people who had forgotten The Quran in their worldly life."*

Everyone in the congregation was quiet, waiting to hear from the imam as to what the one and only reason for Muslim's decline was and what the one and only solution was.

The imam broke his silence and said, "the reason for all the problems Muslims have in today's world is that they do not wear caps, all the time, every time. If you wear caps all the time, all your problems would be solved."

If it were not for the Friday prayer, I would have walked out of the mosque.

I knew this imam very well. He wore a cap all the time, every time, everywhere and yet he had many problems in his life, lots of health issues and other issues. I knew all this because he used to consult me. He was a qualified imam from a well-known religious school in India.

Do we need such fiction? Is this Islam? Is this speaker an Aalim (religious scholar)? The same imam, in another Friday sermon, said about how hard the Aalim course was, and he spent seven years studying this course.

Saying this, I know other imams from the same religious school. They do not say things like this. All though in their sermons they do not discuss contemporary issues, the importance of worldly education, especially science and technology, do say controversial points but within the limits of common sense.

b. Miracle of a four-year-old child.

This is the speech given in a mosque in the UK by a well-known guest speaker during Ramadhan.

In the 16th century, there was a pious, religious couple in Delhi, India. They had a boy. When the boy grew to the age of four, the father took the boy to a saint to teach him about reading the Quran. This was the tradition in those days, i.e., when any child was four years old, he was taken to some teacher/saint to start learning the Quran.

This boy was also taken to the saint. The saint asked the boy to repeat after him the first verse in the first surah (chapter) of the Quran. The boy started reading (verbally) and went on to read fifteen chapters of the Quran, non-stop without looking into the Quran. The saint was amazed. The saint asked him, "How do you know the fifteen chapters of the Quran by heart? You are only four years old?"

The boy replied, "When I was in my mummy's tummy, she used to read Quran, I used to listen and that is how I memorised the fifteen chapters."

This was regarded by the speaker as a miracle.

Comments:

Let us consider what a miracle is? A miracle is a super/unnatural occurrence beyond the capacity of any human being to perform. According to the Quran and other heavenly books, most miracles were performed by the messengers of Allah, by the will of Allah, before a group of people to convince them when they refused to listen to the messenger of Allah.

When this four-year-old boy read fifteen chapters of the Quran, there were only three persons present there, the boy himself, the father of the boy and the saint. So, who was supposed to be 'convinced' by this miracle? All three people present there were Muslims.

The second point is that it takes, for an adult, about four to six hours to read fifteen chapters of the Quran. This four-year-old boy stood for at least four hours, continuously reciting the Quran. He did not feel thirsty, hungry, did not need to go to the washroom, and did not feel tired.

The third point is, does this story have any practical implication? At most, it creates a 'feel good' factor in the audience that "what a great religion Islam is."

Islam is a great religion, but not by such fictional stories.

Do we need such fiction? Is this Islam? Is the speaker a scholar?

c. Grave full of fire.

This is written in a religious book by a 'well-respected' scholar.

A person died. His body was taken to the graveyard. Some people went down into the grave to lay down the body at rest. Among these people who went down into the grave was a person called Hasan (not the real name). After the burial procedure was complete, the grave was covered with wooden slabs, mud and closed.

When Hasan came back to his house, he realised that his wallet was missing. He was sure that it had fallen into the grave when he went down into the grave to put the body at rest. He went back to the graveyard, opened the grave to get his wallet back. He found that the grave was full of fire. The conclusion was that the dead person was having the 'punishment of the grave'.

Comments:

One of the subjects taught in medical school is forensic medicine. One of the chapters in this subject is the exhumation of the dead bodies for investigation purposes. There is a standard procedure for this and almost always, police are involved. Thousands of dead bodies have been exhumed in the world, and not even one has been found burnt unless the person buried in the grave died in a fire.

In our medical school, we used to dissect the dead bodies in the dissection hall. Once the dissection was over, the remains were buried in the backyard of the dissection hall. A few months/years later, the remains were exhumed to get the skeletons out for the teaching purpose. On not a single occasion, any skeleton was found burnt.

Going through the literature, some scholars believe that the punishment of the grave is given to the soul and not to the actual dead body.

The story written above is a pure work of fiction. Whoever does not believe me, can do the following to prove me wrong.

Ask any police force how many bodies they have exhumed so far and how many of these bodies they found, "burnt." Under the freedom of information act, they are obliged to give this information. The answer will be nil (unless the person died in a fire). Even if they found one single burnt body, I will believe every fiction written in this book. This book is regularly read in Asian mosques. I used to sit in those gatherings, but since I was not allowed to raise any objections any questions, I stopped attending those gatherings. I feel sorry for those who sit there, listen to such stories, believe in them, and think what a great religion Islam is. Islam is a great religion, but not by such fictional stories.

Do we need such fiction to show and convince ourselves that Islam is a great religion? Is this Islam?

d. Constipation relieved.

This story is written in the same book as the one above.

Person "A" had a horse who was always constipated. "A" was quite worried about the constipation of his horse. With all the treatments available, there was no positive result, i.e., constipation was not relieved.

One day, "A" was going somewhere on the back of his constipated horse. On the way, at a particular place, suddenly, the horse's constipation was relieved. "A" was surprised. When "A" came back home, again, the horse was constipated and remained constipated for few days until, by chance, "A" was going to the same place as before. Again, at the same place as before, the horse's constipation was relieved. This happened few times. When the horse was at home or anywhere else, it was constipated, but at that particular place, its constipation was relieved. "A" was very surprised. He consulted a 'religious person'. The religious person, along with "A", went to that place, where the horse was relieving its constipation. The religious person looked at the ground for few moments and declared, "There is a person buried here, he is having the punishment of the grave, that is why the horse, whenever it comes here, gets terrified and relieves its constipation."

Is this another fantastic proof of the punishment of the grave?

Is this how Islam should be portrayed? Is this Islam?

Comments:

As I have mentioned above, some scholars believe that the punishment of the grave is given to the soul and not to the dead body.

In India, the graveyards are not looked after as well as here in the UK. Many graves are broken and crumble with time. You can see inside of the grave. There is no evidence of the burnt bodies inside the graves. Many animals roam round in the graveyards. They are not constipated; they are not there to relieve their constipation.

Is this how to make people believe in the punishment of the grave?

Is this Islam?

e. Hanging arm.

A 12-year-old boy was taking part in a battle. He entered the battlefield in the morning. As soon as he entered there, his right arm was severed near the shoulder by an enemy's sword. It was just hanging by a piece of the skin. The boy put that arm at his back and continued fighting till the evening, i.e., for about 7-8 hours.

Comments:

Grown-up, well-built companions of the Prophet (PBUH) have died in the battles, on the spot, when they were hit by arrows or cut by swords. Ameer Hamza (R.A.) died with one throw of the spear and yet, here was a 12-year-old boy, fighting all day with his arm hanging by a piece of skin. His arteries, veins, nerves, bone etc., were cut, yet he was fully conscious and could fight all day. Blood flow through the brachial and circumflex arteries is such that when they are cut, the person loses consciousness very soon and dies within a very short time.

This story and others mentioned in this chapter are supposed to strengthen our 'Imaan', i.e., faith. Do we need such stories to strengthen our faith? Is the Quran not enough for us? People, who write such stories, are they scholars? Is this Islam?

f. 3-1, 1-3 (The Quran has 7339 verses and a single man will take many hours, definitely more than three hours, to read the whole Quran in one sitting.)

Now, here is the story.

There were three very religious, very pious people. They used to 'finish' one Quran each and every night. There was another person, more advanced than these three people. He used to 'finish' three Qurans every night.

Comments:

1. Nowhere in the Quran it says that you finish one Quran or three Qurans in one night.
2. The Prophet (PBUH) never finished one or three Qurans in one night.
3. The maximum, recorded in the literature, is that the Prophet read six parts of the Quran in one night (There are 114 parts in the Quran).
4. In Surah: 73, verses: 2 and 3, Allah is asking the Prophet to reduce the amount of Quran he was reciting in his prayers.
5. In the same Surah, Allah is asking the Prophet (and us) to recite the Quran slowly, peacefully, with clear pronunciation (a second person listing to this recitation should be able to understand what is being recited).
6. It takes about eight to ten hours for one person to recite the whole Quran from the first page to the last page. Our pious people, who recited one Quran every night and three Qurans every night, must be superhumans

to have that much stamina. In any case, where did they find the time to do so? Obviously, they started after the Isha (late night) prayer and had to finish by the morning prayer (dawn time).

7. If this was the routine for them, every night, obviously, they must have been sleeping all day the next day. How did they make their living? What was their productivity? Did they work and contribute to the GDP? Or did they rely on hand outs?

8. Even if it is all true, it has no lesson for common, working men. This is an impractical, unworkable Islam.

9. I say this to the scholars/imams: "say something which the working population can easily do." From the life of the Prophet, we learn that he used to divide the night into three parts. One part was to spend time with the family, another to rest and the third to pray.

10. For the working population, one should read/study a small portion of the Quran every day. Read with meanings and understanding. It should not affect your work the next day; (one doctor was warned for his behaviour. He was found dozing off to sleep while he was supposed to look after patients. The reason he was dozing off was that he was spending too much time at night, in prayers and reading Quran). Your work and your 'rights/obligations to others' should not be affected by your night prayers. You are paid for the work you do. Make this payment 'Halal' by doing your job properly.

11. Read those parts of the Quran first, which give 'rules, regulations and principles' of life. For example, Surah: 3, Verses: 190-193, Surah: 23, verses: 1-11, Surah: 25, Verses: 63-77, and many more. They form the, "Principles and practice of life…an Islamic perspective."

Such verses are scattered all over the Quran. This is an incentive for the reader to go through the whole Quran, although you can get the basic message of the Quran by reading a small portion.

In any religion, there are six things:

a) Concept of God.
b) Other beliefs.
c) Its rituals.
d) General principles.

e) Specific principles.

f) How does it persuade its followers to follow its principles?

The Quran not only gives principles of life but also puts many arguments, reasoning, logic, intelligent thinking, examples, and historical evidence to persuade its followers to put the principles into practice. These are scattered throughout the Quran. The fundamentals are very simple:

1. There is only one God. 2. You are responsible and accountable for your actions. 3. We all return to Allah. 4. Resurrection Day i.e., the Day of Judgement is a reality and WILL come; there is no doubt about it.

g) Riding a tiger:

In a village (where? God knows.), the farmers were working in the fields. They saw a man with a turban, beard and typical Muslim appearance riding along the fields on a tiger. The villagers were amazed. They asked him how he managed to ride a tiger. The man answered, Allah, said in the Quran, "We have subdued, for you, what is in the heavens and on the earth." This was his explanation of being able to ride a tiger.

Comments:

This verse that says, "Allah has subdued for you (Man) what is in the heavens and in the earth," appears in many places in the Quran, e.g., Surah 31, verse 20, Surah 45, verses 3 and 12. This means that everything in the heavens and earth is working for the benefit of 'Man' by Allah's will. For example, the sun, moon, stars, wind, clouds, rain etc. This does not mean that man has control over wild animals.

In another place, in the Quran, Surah 36, verses 71-73, Allah says that He has made the domestic animals for your benefits and subdued them for you. Some you use for food, some you ride, and there are other benefits as well.

The writer of this story has misunderstood the interpretation of these verses and made the story. All the people who say such 'unnatural, miraculous' things in their speeches, I ask them, "have you, yourself witnessed any such miracle?" The answer is always, 'No'. It is always heard and said with lots of exaggeration and twisting. It is very easy to fool people in the name of religion.

Do we need such fiction to strengthen our faith (Imaan)? Is this Islam?

h) One ablution and 12 days prayer.

Ablution is the process of washing one's hands, forearms, cleaning the nose, face, head, and feet before performing any prayer. There are certain things which break the ablution, for example, if the person goes to the toilet to pass urine or to open his bowels, etc., He must do another ablution before he could pray.

A guest speaker in a mosque in London said that a man was so pious, so religious, so devoted to his prayers that he used to perform twelve days' worth of prayers (praying five times a day) with one ablution.

Comments:

This means he did not use the toilet for 12 days, i.e., did not pass urine and did not open his bowels, for 12 days. He did not even pass wind through his back passage for 12 days.

Laws of nature do not change for anyone regardless of how religious and pious the person is. This theme is in the Quran in many places. If this person did not pass urine for 12 days, his serum potassium should have been so high and other biochemistry should have been so abnormal that he should have been seriously ill or even dead.

How did people know that he was doing 12 days of prayers with one ablution?

Looking at a person, can you tell if he has or has not passed urine? Has or has not opened his bowels? Unless this pious man himself went around telling people, "Look, I am so pious, and this is what I am doing. My last ablution was 12 days ago."

Do we need such fiction? Is this Islam? By saying such stories, what are they, our scholars, trying to prove? Are they scholars or 'story tellers'?

i. One Quran in one Rakat.

A Rakat is a unit of prayer. One unit contains four parts; the first part (Qiyam) is done in a standing position when the worshiper recites a portion of the Quran. This is usually the longest part of the Rakat.

In a gathering, in a mosque, after the evening prayers, a book was read. This is what it said:

One person was, again, so religious, so pious that he used to finish reciting one whole Quran in each one Rakat of each prayer of the day.

Comments:

a) Reading the Quran from the 1ˢᵗ page to the last page takes 8-12 hours. The minimum number of Rakats, in a prayer, are two. Therefore, this person was spending at least 16 hours in one prayer, and he must have been standing in one place, without moving for at least 8 hours in each Rakat.

The total number of Rakats in the five daily obligatory prayers are 17. If this person was reciting one Quran in each Rakat, taking at least 8 hours for each Rakat, then his day must have been at least 136 hours. When did he eat, drink, sleep, go for natural needs? Was he working? Earning his own living, or was he relying on handouts?

b) The Prophet (PBUH) never finished one Quran in one Rakat.

c) Nor there is a hadith to do so.

d) In fact, when the Prophet was reciting the Quran for longer hours of the night, he was told to shorten the recitation; surah 73, verses 2-4.

e) In verse 4 of the above surah (73), Allah says to recite the Quran clearly, meaning words should be pronounced clearly and stop at the end of sentences. If a second person is listening to this recitation, he should be able to clearly hear the words.

By finishing one Quran in each Rakat, the above requirements are not fulfilled. In fact, this person was going against the commands of the Quran.

f) Nowhere in the Quran, Allah says to finish one Quran in one Rakat.

Again, do we need such fiction? What are they, our so-called scholars, trying to prove? Is this Islam?

g) No Qiya'mah (Resurrection Day in London).

A lady, who I know personally, told me that when she was leaving Hyderabad, India, for good, to come to London, she went to say a final goodbye to her murshid (religious teacher). When the teacher heard that she was going to

London, he told her that it was a very good move as there won't be any resurrection and therefore no Judgement Day in London.

Comments:

a) Does this teacher know anything about Islam? Has he read the Quran?

b) Sometimes, these religious teachers say what pleases their followers. This way, their bread and butter keep coming in. They know that they (the religious teachers) can say anything they like, and the followers will believe it. They know the psychology of Muslims that "Muslims do not think. You can say whatever you want, they will believe, blindly," as this lady did.

c) Blind belief in our religious 'leaders' is a big problem within Asian communities. What people do not realise is that when they stand in front of Allah on the Day of Resurrection, they will be on their own. These religious teachers, leaders, muftis, will not be there to rescue them. This is the theme in many places in the Quran. For example, the following verse:

"Oh believers, take care of your own selves (guard your own souls). If you follow the right **guidance**, no harm will come to you from those who are in error. The return of you all is to Allah and He will inform you of all which you did."
Surah: 5, Verse: 105.

Here, "guidance," means the Quran and authentic Ahadees (Prophetic sayings).

We read the first chapter of the Quran in every prayer. One of the verses we read is.

"*Show us the right path.*" If you are sincere in your prayers, Allah will always keep you on the right path. However, there is one more prayer that is not in Quran, but the Prophet (PBUH) used to say this prayer very frequently and that is:

"Oh, our Lord, show us the truth as truth and inspire us to follow it and show us the falsehood as falsehood and inspire us to avoid it."

With this in mind, whatever your religious teacher says, you will be able to work out what is the truth.

h) Wolf and the goat:

This story was read from a religious book after the evening prayers. It is claimed to be true.

There was a king in Iraq. He was so fair and just that in his kingdom, a wolf and a goat drank water, side by side, from the same river. The king lived in Bagdad, the capital city of Iraq.

One day, an old woman, who was hundreds of miles away from Bagdad, was watching the river from her house. She saw a wolf drinking water from the river. Then a goat came to drink the water. The wolf attacked the goat and killed it.

The woman came out of her house and started shouting: "The king is dead; the king is dead." People asked her how she knew that king was dead as she was hundreds of miles away from Bagdad. She said that she saw a wolf killing a goat, and this was the sign that the king was dead.

Comments:

1. What a wonderful story…to prove what?
2. If the king was so fair that the wolf and the goat drank water from the same river at the same time, i.e., the wolf did not kill the goat for its food, I would say that the king was so unfair and cruel that in his kingdom, wolves went hungry.
3. Allah has set certain rules to run this world. They form 'laws of nature'. One such law is, "One life has to be destroyed, in order for the other life to survive." We eat meat and eggs. We are destroying other lives to survive. Plants have life. We eat fruits and vegetables. We are destroying other lives.
4. It is a phrase in the Urdu language that if a ruler is very fair and just, it is said, "in his kingdom, wolf and goat drink water from the same river, at the same time." It does not mean this literally happens; it is just a way of expressing fairness and justice.

I remember reading history books in Hyderabad, India, in the 1950s. In these books, King Ashoka the great, King Akbar the great and King Jahangir were described in this way. The writer of the above story is not an Urdu speaking person; therefore, he took the phrase literally and made the story.

201

Note:

Certain phrases of the old Arabic language are used in the Quran. We need to be careful in their interpretation. For this purpose, I refer to 'Arab' Qurans and not the 'Asian' Qurans. Arab Qurans mean, Quranic translation and explanation written by Arabs. It is their language; they know it better.

Examples of such verses are Surah: 11, verse: 107, Surah: 7, verse: 40, Surah: 5, verse 45 etc.

When studying the Quran, keep an open mind. If you do not understand any verse or its explanation, look into other books or ask people with knowledge. This concept of 'ask people of knowledge' is from the Quran.

1. TV girl:

This is written in one of the so-called Islamic literatures. The book was printed in India, written by a well-known 'scholar'. I found the book in my local mosque. People leave books of their liking in the mosque for other people to read/take home. They think that this is a great service to their Muslim brothers.

While most books are fine, some are not.

Here is the story from the book. I found it hilarious. The writer says it to be true.

A teenage Muslim girl was very fond of television. It was her routine that every day, after coming back from school, she would watch TV for some time.

It was Ramadhan; the girl came back from school and shut herself in her room, watching TV. Her mother called her for help in the kitchen. The girl did not go to the kitchen. When the time came to break the fast (iftar), the mother called the girl, but the girl did not reply. After few calls, the mother went to the girl's room. She found the girl dead. The TV was on. The mother and the family were very sad. The funeral was arranged a few days later. The girl's body was taken to the graveyard, and it was buried. The next day, somebody came from the graveyard and said that the grave was found opened and the girl's body was lying on the ground, outside the grave. The family went to the graveyard, thought that an enemy must have done this, and reburied the body. The next day again, the girl's body was found outside the grave. This continued for few days. The family approached their Murshid (religious teacher). The teacher asked about the girl's routine. When he heard that the girl used to watch TV every day, he said to the family that unless they bury the TV with her body in the grave, this would keep happening. The family, very obediently, buried the TV with the girl's body. The end of the story was that the family returned home 'happy ever after'.

Analysis: What a wonderful way of stopping people from watching TV. People who write such fiction are totally ignorant of their surroundings and especially ignorant of the needs of the younger generation. Instead of asking them to stop watching TV, teach them right and wrong. This way, they will not watch 'nudity' but will get all the benefits of scientific, political, social programmes and news. The previous imam of the local mosque used to watch TV and used to discuss 'Question times' with me. The present imam of my hospital watches all the useful programmes, he is up to date with what is happening in the world and his Friday sermons are always focused on current affairs.

The person who wrote the above story, is he really an Islamic scholar, as claimed in the book, or is he a good storyteller? Is this Islam?

m. How to identify…

This I found on YouTube.

Sometimes, police in the villages in Pakistan find some unclaimed dead bodies. Probably these are homeless, poor people without families. It becomes the police's responsibility to conduct their funerals. As there is some non-Muslim population there as well, the police have to identify if the dead person is Muslim or non-Muslim. With male bodies, the job is very easy. Muslims' bodies are circumcised. However, if the body is that of a female, then it becomes a problem. The Police have no way of finding if the dead women are Muslims or non-Muslims.

So, the police approached a 'religious person', well-known in the villages, for his 'knowledge of Islam'. He said, "give a bath to the dead woman, collect the water of the bath and put it in front of a horse. If the horse drinks the water, then the body is that of a Muslim woman."

Analysis: No analysis as it is a waste of time to do so. This sort of fiction gives Islam nothing but a bad name.

n. Sermon for the prayer on Friday, 19 May 2017.

Ramadhan was in 8 days' time. The Imam started saying the importance of reading the Quran, especially in the month of Ramadhan. This was fine, no objection. Then the Imam said:

a) Imam Abu-Hanifa (R.A.) used to read the entire Quran (7339 verses) 61 times every Ramadhan. One during the day, every day, second at night, every night, and the third in the Taraweeh prayer. Note: To read the complete Quran from page 1 to the last page takes 8-12 hours, at least.

b) b). Shah Ismail Shaheed (R.A.) of India used to finish one Quran every day between Asar and Maghrib prayers. The time gap between Asar and Maghrib prayer is usually 2-3 hours.

I caught the Imam next day and asked him a few questions:

Q1. It takes about 8-12 hours for one person to finish reading the Quran, from page 1 to the last page. How did these two people finish reading the entire Quran in such a short period?

Answer: It was a miracle.

Q2. Not a single book on the life of the Prophet (PBUH) says that he used to read the entire Quran, 61 times in the month of Ramadhan, or one Quran every day between Asar and Maghrib prayers (about 3 hours). Does this mean that these two persons have a higher position than the Prophet?

Answer: No, the reason is that if he (the Prophet) would have done like these two persons, then it would have become an obligation for the Muslims to do so.

What this Imam forgot is that the Prophet did quite a few things in his lifetime, due to his special position or due to circumstances, which are not obligatory for Muslims to do. For example, he wrote letters to the rulers/kings of various nations, inviting them to Islam. Do all the Muslims have to write letters to some kings and queens? This is just one example. There are many others.

Q3. You regard this as a miracle, yes? "Yes," he replied. You have mentioned other miracles of the 'friends of Allah'. Have you personally witnessed any miracle from these people?

Answer: "No...but it is written in books."

Q4. Is there any mention of 'miracles of friends of Allah' in the Quran or Ahadees (Prophet's sayings)?

Answer: "No."

Q5. Muslims who do not believe in what you have said about these two people mentioned above, are these Muslims committing any sin by not believing in your stories?

Answer: "No."

Q6. In Surah 73, verse 4, Allah asks the Muslims to recite the Quran, slowly and clearly. The Prophet used to recite it slowly and clearly and he asked us, the Muslims, to do so. By not doing so, did these two persons, in your story, not go against the Quran and the Sunnah?

Answer: "Yes, but it is a miracle."

Q7. What these two persons did, if true, has no lesson for common, working Muslims. So, what was the purpose of mentioning these two stories?

Answer: "To persuade Muslims to read more Quran."

Comments:

What a wonderful, unbelievable, impractical, unworkable Islam.

I have heard many of our 'religious' speakers mentioning all kinds of miracles of the 'Friends of Allah'. None of them have personally witnessed any such miracle. This is all word of mouths, spread over the centuries, with lots of lies, exaggerations, twisting etc., by the devotees of that particular 'Friend of Allah'.

Imams and other speakers should say something which is workable and practical for a common man. Say something which makes sense.

I narrated these two stories to few people and asked them, "Do these stories persuade you to read more Quran?" Everyone said, "No," with one lady saying that such stories would put her off from the Quran and the religion. I do not blame any one of them. If our religious leaders/imams are like this, then it is hard to believe that our religion is the right religion.

While the rest of the world is doing miracles by advancing in science and technology, reaching the moon and Mars, we, the Muslims, are doing miracles by believing in such stories. This is because we have a blind belief in our so-called scholars.

Once I overheard one person saying to the other person, "If you want to understand Islam, keep away from Asian scholars." No matter how much I hate to believe in this, but when I hear such stories written in this chapter, I intend to believe that the man was right.

Once, someone said, "The miracle of Islam is that its followers believe in everything given to them, in the name of their religion, by their scholars."

We need an overhaul in our understanding of Islam.

All the people (scholars) who have written the stories which I have collected in this chapter have also written good, sensible articles on various Islamic topics.

It is still a mystery to me that why, on one side, these scholars write such nice, decent, and sensible articles and on the other side they write what I have collected in this chapter, i.e., totally unbelievable, impractical, unworkable 'stories' with no sense in it.

How many of us, after reading this chapter, will try to read one Quran between Asar and Maghrib prayer? The answer is none.

How many of us will try to do 12 days of prayers with one ablution? The answer is none.

I used to think that it is their training in religious schools. But then I cannot explain: **a)** why all of them are not like this? The religious schools have produced some very good, sensible scholars.

b) I am surprised to find some educated people, like doctors, engineers, architects etc., who have not been to any religious schools, and yet they believe and speak in favour of the stories which I have written in this chapter. Therefore, religious schools are not always to be blamed.

c) Some well-educated, well-known people who have never been to a religious school yet gained the knowledge by self-studies. They never say any unbelievable, impractical, and unworkable, senseless stories like those mentioned in this chapter. Why are they not like people in group b?

My personal view/explanation is that:

a)   Whether a human being uses his intelligence or not?

b)   Whether he uses his ability to think, reason, logic or not?

c)   Whether he knows his limits or not?

d)   Most importantly, whether he understands the Quran or not? Whether he grasps the fundamentals from it or not? And finally, whether he uses these principles with common sense or not.

o. In his book "Tarashey", published in June 2014 in Karachi, Pakistan; Mufti Taqi Usmani quotes some 'true stories' which are unbelievable and have no practical importance:

1. On pages 75 and 76, he quotes that Abdullah-bin-Mubarak (R.A.) was a pious person. However, he was not like this from the beginning. He was very much into wine, women, and music. One night he drank a lot of alcohol. In the morning, when he got up, he picked up his musical instrument and started to play. The instrument did not play; instead, a sound came from the instrument and said," Is this not the right time for people to subdue their hearts to Allah?"

However, Taqi Usmani Sahib also writes that this incidence is narrated by another historian in a different way, i.e., Abdullah-bin Mubarak, in his dream, saw an animal sitting on a tree and reciting this verse from the Quran.

By quoting the two different versions of the story, he has created a lot of doubts. More importantly, this has no bearing, no lesson for a common working Muslim in the 21st century.

2. On pages 77 and 78, he writes that Rabi bin Hirash (R.A.) and his brother Raba'ee bin Harish (R.A.) were very pious people. They both vowed that until they knew how they would be treated after their death, they won't laugh. All their life, they did not laugh.

After their death, when the bodies were being cleaned and bathed, they started laughing.

They had another brother, Masood (R.A.). Apparently, he talked to people after his death.

These are just the two examples. There are some more unbelievable incidences like this.

What I do not understand is that if all these people, whom I mentioned in this chapter, were so great, pious people, showing all kinds of miracles, why did they not keep Islam simple? Why did they not say to the people that Islam is very simple and straightforward? Study the Quran, understand the fundamentals, put them into practice and get on with life?

I think the above incidences, where dead people talked/laughed, were simply a matter of rigour mortis, which affects the facial muscles as well. The narrator has exaggerated the whole incidence to make it look like a miracle.

As a teenager in India, it was my duty to go and buy fresh meat from the butcher's shop every morning before going to school. I noticed many times that the leg of the lamb was hanging in the shop and from time to time, it was contracting. The animal had been slaughtered some time ago and the rest of its body was somewhere else.

Later, as a medical student, I learnt about the physiology of the muscle and knew the reason for the contraction in the legs of the lambs.

Death has stages, clinical death, biological death and cellular death. Even after the 'death' of a person/animal, some parts/organs of the body are functioning, for some time, under reduced conditions, i.e., less oxygen etc. The brain of a dead person is alive for some time after the clinical death and hearing is the last sensation to go. A dying/ dead person can hear you for some time, although he may not understand it. The same is true for a patient having general anaesthetics for operation. Hearing is the last sensation to go under anaesthetics and first to come back, as the patient wakes up from anaesthetics. There have been some unpleasant incidences in the operation theatres due to this.

Coming back to our miraculous people who laughed and talked after their death, I have explained the reason, in my view, of their, what looked like laughing.

As to the talking, the air in the stomach of a dead person can flow up and come out from the mouth as a sound. I have noticed this many times in my medical practice in the recently dead and unconscious patients. This is one of the reasons that all dead people's s orifices are blocked by cotton wool. In the story above, the narrator has exaggerated the event.

I have heard many times the speakers, and scholars of Islam, talking about the 'Miracles of the Saints' (karamat-e-Awliya). I asked them, "Have you, yourself, witnessed any of the miracles you mentioned in your speech?" The answer has always been, "No." For the speakers, it is simply a matter of hear and say, believe in it, make people believe and thus make Islam a great religion…"Look, we have such great saints." These speeches and writings by the so-called scholars are nothing but good entertainment. They simply create a false feel-good factor in the audience. The audience comes out of the mosque thinking what a great religion Islam is.

If we have such great miracle performing saints, why can't they join forces and perform the miracle of the century, i.e., persuade Donald Trump to reverse his decision about Jerusalem? (In the year 2017, Trump has recognised Jerusalem as the capital of Israel). The entire Muslim world is unhappy about this decision, but it cannot do anything about it. Where are our "Miracle performing saints"?

I have, and I still do, read 'Islamic literature'. There are two words I love to find in this literature, but so far have failed to find them. These two words are: **Science and Technology**. The future saints performing miracles will be the scientists.

There is nothing new in this world except what we don't know.

Unexplained things do have an explanation. We call them unexplained because we do not know the mechanism of their action.

A mobile phone (cell phone), a TV, an aeroplane etc., are not miracles because we know how they work. If you give these things to someone who has never seen them before, they will regard these things as 'Miracles'. I remembered in 1956, when we first bought our 'radio' in the village, some older people recognised it as a miracle. Some said that there was a jinn inside the box talking and singing and giving the latest news.

Use the God-given gift, i.e., thinking, reasoning and logic. Know your limits.

p) Recently (October 2018), I read a book in Urdu. The title is: "For children, interesting and lessons to learn Islamic stories.", by Aleem publishers, Gadhafi stadium, Urdu Bazar, Lahore 2 Pakistan. 1st printed 1984.

On page 14, it says, "Saint Bayazeed Batami was having difficulties in getting up at night to do his prayers. He realised that it was his physical desires which were preventing him from doing so. So, to kill his physical desires, he decided not to drink water for one year and he did so."

Is this Islam? Is this Islamic teaching? What lessons do children learn from this?

Similar stories were there on pages 21 and 72.

My only comment is, what nonsense. If a person does not drink water, he dies in 7-10 days. The First 3-4 days, he is conscious, though disorientated, weak, and lethargic, then he loses consciousness, goes into a coma and dies.

Q. As per imam of my local mosque, London E11, another 'great Muslim saint', to control his physical desires, did not sleep, with his back to his bed, for one year.

Comment: Pure fib. No lesson to be learnt.

R. One more miracle by a wonderful saint.

In the 1965 war between India and Pakistan, Indian fighter planes went to Pakistani territory to bomb.

The people on the ground, in the Pakistani territory, saw that as the bombs were falling, an old man with a long white beard with a very sacred lit up face (lit up with the light of God) flew in the air, collected all the bombs, thrown by the Indian Airforce, brought them back to the earth, gave it to the Pakistani air force and they were used against India.

This is the miracle our saints do, and we believe. This story was told by an outside speaker, a 'learn-ed' man, in my local mosque.

It is nothing but nonsense. Unfortunately, most people attending the mosque believe such stories. All I can say that Muslims are very easily fooled by such stories. This is because they have no idea what God has given to them.

Chapter Twenty-One
Funny Side of Hospital Work (40 True Stories)

Working in hospitals is a serious business. We are surrounded by sick people, people in pain, terminally ill patients, patients having routine and emergency surgeries, women delivering babies with or without complications, anxious and worried patients and their relatives, children with their anxious parents, patients dying in front of your eyes, seriously ill patients in the ICU and in the resuscitation room, etc. We switch off the ventilators (breathing machines) on brain dead patients, we write DNR (do not resuscitate) orders, etc.

Once, I had a patient who was due to have an emergency surgery. I told the relatives to let the patient die peacefully because, in my opinion, that patient was going to die anyway, with or without surgery, so why put him through a painful procedure. The team, including the consultant surgeon, agreed with my decision. The relatives agreed as well. The patient died a few hours later, peacefully.

Once I was on call for the night. At 2 a.m., a consultant gynaecologist rang me. His wordings were: "Khan, come quickly; I have a dying patient in my hand."

I jumped into my car. Halfway to the hospital, that consultant rang and said: "No need to come, the patient has died."

This is the life of doctors who work in acute specialities.

Sometimes doctors feel that it is better if the patient dies rather than survive. I have seen this when I was doing my neurosurgical work as a junior doctor. With brain trauma, some patients survive but become mentally or physically disabled or go into a vegetative state, i.e., they are alive but disorientated. They do not know who they are, where they are, what is the day and date, cannot recognise their relatives etc. They are just alive. In Hyderabad, in the 1960s, one patient, in a vegetative state, lived for eleven years. There was no concept of mercy killing in those days. I have seen disabled children due to brain trauma at birth.

Fortunately, by 2017/18, thanks to all the scientists and researchers, mainly in the West, medicine has advanced to such an extent that what I had seen as a trainee has become a thing of the past. The outcome for stroke patients is far better now than it used to be 40-50 years ago.

Some of the drugs and instruments which I used as a junior doctor have become so 'old' that they are in the museum in the basement of the Royal College of Anaesthetists in London, labelled as 'Obsolete anaesthetic drugs and instruments'.

Saying all this, the hospitals are very safe places. The staff are highly skilled and trained, highly qualified, and very efficient, very conscious of their duties. The vast majority of patients go home safely.

Despite the serious work we do get from time to time, some funny stories. Here are some of them I personally came across. They are all true. Names of people and places have been changed.

These true stories should be taken lightly. They are not meant to hurt anyone's feelings or degrade or make fun of anyone. Values and views change with time. What was 'funny' 40/45 years ago maybe a 'sensitive' issue today. So, see them as old-fashioned funny stories.

1. Do you eat halal meat?

I was working in a hospital in Kent. As I had to do night duties as well, I looked forward to my nights off. Once, after working all day in the operation theatres, I came home around at 6 p.m. I was off that night. I went to bed around 10 p.m. Around 2 a.m., the phone rang. The person on the other side said to me, "Dr Khan, can you please come to the theatres immediately." I told him that I was off duty, and he needed to call the duty doctor. The person on the phone said that the matter was something very different and he requested me to come to the theatres as soon as possible. So, I want to the theatres. The story was as follows: It was a Muslim female patient who needed an emergency Caesarean section to save her baby. She insisted that at least one doctor in the team should be a Muslim who eats halal meat. As I approached her, she asked me only one question: "Do you eat halal meat?" After my, "yes," we immediately proceeded with the surgery.

To date, I don't know the connection between halal meat and anaesthetics.

2. I am pregnant

I had a seven-year-old girl with appendicitis. While talking to her, I asked her what did she think was wrong with her? She said, "I am pregnant." I asked her how she knew that she was pregnant. She said, "When my little sister was in my mummy's tummy, my mum used to complain of pain in her tummy. Now I have pain in my tummy, so I must be pregnant."

3. Shall I show you?

An eight-year-old boy was brought to the hospital with broken bones of his left forearm. He was playing with his older sister, who was 11 and she probably hit her brother with a wooden stick so hard that the arm broke. I asked the sister: "How did you manage to break his arm?" She said: "Very easily, shall I show you on his other arm?"

4. Patient cleaned with her urine

It was a gynaecological operating session. The patient was anaesthetised and was on the operating table. The consultant gynaecologist walked in, asked her assistant to "'prepare' the patient, which included catheterisation of the urinary bladder and draping. The assistant catheterised the patient and left the urine in a kidney tray near the patient. The consultant walked in, thought that the urine was Savalon (a cleaning liquid that is yellow in colour) and started cleaning the patient's abdomen with the urine. Those who knew that it was urine shouted, "Oh, Miss…, this is the patient's urine." Then she stopped. Fortunately, such mistakes are very rare, especially after the introduction of the WHO checklist (WHO checklist is a method of checking all the details about the operation a patient is going to have, including the instruments, etc.).

5. Send the patient with...

In an orthopaedic operating theatre, the consultant surgeon told his assistant to ring the ward to send for the next patient. The next patient was due to have surgery on his left leg. The assistant was from a non-English speaking country. He rang the ward and said to the nurse, "This is theatres. Please send the next patient with his left leg."

6. "Dr Khan...please..."

I was working in Saudi Arabia. Most of the nurses were from the far East. One night, a nurse from the ward rang me and said, "Oh, Dr Khan, the patient in bed No 22 has not passed urine for the last 12 hours. Please come and pass some urine."

7. Broken heart

In the same hospital, the routine was that the patient's final diagnosis was written in one or two words on the front page of the notes. A patient who had mitral valve incompetence (a defective valve in the heart) was admitted. The diagnosis on the front page was written as 'Broken heart'.

8. Good morning Mr... Good evening Miss...

I was the consultant anaesthetist in a sex change operation where a man was to be converted into a woman.

My assistant started writing his notes as "He is fit and healthy. His blood results are fine. His blood pressure, pulse and other parameters are fine." Towards the end of the surgery, she (my assistant) started writing, "She (the patient) is fine. She is waking up nicely. Her pulse and BP are fine."

In the morning, when we saw the patient in the ward, my assistant greeted him as "Hello, Mr..." In the evening, after the surgery, when we saw the patient again in the recovery room of the operation theatres, my assistant said, "Hello, Madam..."

What a change a few hours can make. *No offence to LGBT or anyone.*

9. Small>>>>Big>>>>small. (No offence to anyone)

This happened to one of my colleagues:

A young woman came to him for the augmentation of her breasts. When asked why she wanted to have implants in her breasts. She said that her breasts were small, and her boyfriend did not like small breasts. The operation was done. She had implants in her breasts.

About a year later, she came and said that she wanted the implants removed. When asked why she wanted them removed, she said, "I have changed my boyfriend, and he does not like big breasts." *No offence to anyone.*

10. Push...Push. No...you pull.

Women in labour wards are encouraged to 'push' when delivering babies. It is common for nurses and doctors to keep saying "push...push...push..."

In a private hospital, a woman was delivering her baby. She was told to, "push...push...push again." She got angry and said, "I am a private patient; why should I push? ...you pull."

11. Will you...?

In the 1970s, I was working in Harrogate, Yorkshire as a junior doctor. I had a 13-year-old girl for abdominal surgery. I looked after her before and after her operation. Her recovery was uneventful. I reported back to my consultant that she was well and could be discharged. The consultant told me to go and discharge her and write the discharge notes.

I went to the ward, wrote the discharge notes and the letter and gave them to the nurses. I told the patient that she could go home.

An hour later, I got a call from the ward to go there urgently. I thought, OMG! I must have made some mistakes. I went to the ward and asked the nurses what the matter was. They told me that the girl wanted to speak to me, and she was not telling anyone, including her parents, what she wanted to speak to me about. She was not going to go home without seeing me. I got worried. I was new in the country and probably said or did something which I should not have done.

I went to see the girl and in the presence of nurses and her parents she told me, "I like you very much, will you marry me?"

12. I do not want to be the president of America...please

I was working in the A & E in a Kent hospital. One night when I was off duty, my phone rang around midnight. The A & E charge nurse told me to come to A & E urgently. I told him that I was off that night, but the charge nurse told me that he had spoken to the consultant on call and the consultant told the charge nurse to call me.

I went to the A & E. The doctor who was supposed to come on duty that night was there but very drunk. He was wandering around in the department shouting, "I do not want to be the president of America, please...I beg you not to elect me."

Between the charge nurse and me, we decided that I would take this doctor to his residence and then I would come and do the night shift.

I asked that doctor where his room was. He said, "room 6, residence 16," In the middle of the night, I took him there and that turned out to be a nurse's home. A nurse from room 6 came out in her nightgown. Then I realised that probably it was the other way round. I took him to residence 6 and dropped him in his room, i.e., room 16. I came back and did the night shift in the A & E.

Obviously, that doctor was reported to the manager the next day.

13. Are you the angel of death?

It was a December night. Around 3 a.m., I was called for a caesarean section. In the theatres, I was in the blue theatres' clothes. I saw the patient, talked to her. She was very scared to go through the operation. She was convinced that she was going to die. She described to me how, in her imagination, the angel of death looked like. It was a shadowy figure in white clothes. I assured her, calmed her down and said that I would be with her throughout the operation and in the recovery room.

She had general anaesthetics. The operation was uneventful. She was taken to the recovery room. As it was around 4:30 a.m. in December, it was getting very cold. I was feeling cold in my theatre blues, so I went to the changing room and put on my white coat. Then I went to the recovery room to see if the patient was fully awake. I was standing next to her, in my white coat. As she started emerging from the anaesthetics, she looked at me and started screaming. Earlier she had seen me in the theatre blues, and now I was standing next to her in my white coat. She thought I was the angel of death and had come to take her soul. She kept asking: "Are you the angel of death? Have you taken my soul? Am I dead?" I remembered how she had described the angel of death…a shadowy white figure. As she was coming out of the general anaesthetics, her vision was a bit hazy and I, in my white coat, became the angel of death. The first thing I did was to take off my white coat. Then it took the nurses and me quite a few minutes to convince her (the patient) that she was not dead. We showed her, her baby. Then it was a happy ending for her and for us.

14. Sorry…I am in Israel

In an afternoon session in a London hospital, the obstetric registrar was doing an elective caesarean section. Halfway through, he got into trouble and wanted the consultant obstetrician urgently. I asked him the name of the on-call consultant obstetrician and then rang the switchboard to call him. A few minutes later, the consultant obstetrician answered. I explained the situation and asked him to come to the theatre immediately. He said, "Sorry I can't come, I am in Israel." Apparently, he went on annual leave but forgot to arrange a cover for himself. Luckily, it was daytime, and many people were available to help. We manage to get another consultant obstetrician, and no harm came to the mother or the baby.

15. Sorry, but she is...

One of my juniors was working in a different theatre. After the surgery, he took the patient to recovery. He expected the patient to wake up after few minutes. When she, the patient, did not wake up, he started saying in a loud voice: "Janet, wake up, your operation is finished." He did this a few times, but Janet still did not wake up. My junior asked me to come to the recovery to find out why the patient was not waking up. It is quite a serious thing if a patient does not wake up after the operation. I went to the recovery, looked at the notes and the monitors. I could not find any reason for the patient not to wake up. I also said, "Janet, wake up your operation is done." She still did not wake up. I called her again...still no response. Then a nurse who was standing nearby said: "Why are you calling her Janet? She is not Janet. She is Betty." I called again, "Betty, open your eyes; your operation is done." She opened her eyes immediately. I asked her if she did not hear my assistant or me. She answered, "Yes, I have heard from the beginning, but I thought you were calling some other patient named Janet."

16. Sorry, but I missed...

In an orthopaedic theatre, the consultant orthopaedic surgeon was trying a new procedure on the patient's leg. As it was a new procedure, which the consultant had read in a journal, he asked his assistant to stand next to him and read the journal while he was operating. After about forty minutes into the surgery, the consultant told his assistant: "I don't think things are going the right way. If I continue like this, the patient will have his leg at a right angle to his thigh. Are you sure you have read correctly?" The assistant looked at the journal again and said, "Sorry sir, but I missed one page." The correct procedure was done, and no harm came to the patient.

17. Talk to me, I am...

In the A & E department, I was doing the night shift. A girl in her twenties was brought in by the ambulance around 3 a.m. She called the ambulance because she got into a panicky state. I called her in my office and asked her about her problem. She said she was very lonely and wanted someone to talk to her. At 3 a.m., I had a general chat with her for about twenty minutes and she was cured of loneliness and panicky state. This happened in a Kent hospital in the 1970s. At that time, I did not realise loneliness was a problem.

Now in 2021, after a lot of experience of life and reading books on psychology and seeing documentaries on loneliness, Covid-19 causing loneliness due to the 'Lockdown' and a 'minister for loneliness' appointed; it is a fact that loneliness can be quite depressive and can create suicidal thoughts. According to one documentary, in northern European countries, the suicide rate among older people is highest in winter when the nights are long. In other news **(B.B.C., 13/04/2017**, a.m., the red button service), loneliness among children in the UK is going up with more girls feeling lonely.

There are verses in the Quran which encourage people to keep in touch with each other and not to break relations. I am sure the books of other religions have similar verses.

18. Did anyone in your family...?

We were in the 3rd year of medicine, where we start out 'clinicals', i.e., we go to the wards and see the real patients.

In the medical wards, we were taught how to take the history from the patients. One of the questions we were supposed to ask was, "Did anyone in your family, in your blood relations, suffer from the same disease as you are suffering now?" This question was to find out about familial diseases like Diabetes, Angina etc., diseases that pass to the next generation through the genes.

After finishing the posting in the medical wards, we went to the orthopaedic and trauma wards. One of my class fellows had a young man, about 17 years old, who fell from a tree and broke his leg. Completely forgetting that he was in a trauma ward, he asked the patient, "Did anyone in your blood relations fall from the tree?" This left us laughing and patient confused.

19. "Oh, Sister...Can't I have...?"

In a London hospital, I was on call for the night. It was my routine that whenever I was on call for the night, I went to the wards around midnight, made sure that everything was alright and then came back to my room to sleep.

In one of the wards, I saw that all the patients had gone to sleep except an old man who was sitting in a deck chair next to his bed. I asked the sister why he was not in his bed; it was midnight. The Sister said, "Let us go and ask him." So, we went to him and the sister asked him, "George, it is midnight; why are you not in your bed?" George answered: "Oh Sister, can't I have some rest before I go to bed?"

This was probably due to the side effects of his medications or the residual effects of the general anaesthetics.

20. ...and fools do not...

A good working relationship without being exploited is important when working with other people. One of the sisters in charge of a ward, sister J, was quite free with me.

A junior doctor, Dr K, was looking at a new admission in sister J's ward. When he finished, he gave the sister in charge 'a diagnosis and a treatment regimen'. She was not happy with the doctor's diagnosis and treatment regimen. She called me for a second opinion. This was not my patient. I had nothing to do with him. However, because the sister and I were on good terms and on many occasions helped each other, I went to the ward and saw the patient. In my view, Dr K was right. I told the sister that Dr K's diagnosis and treatment was right. Dr K was standing there as well. He proudly said to the sister: "See, Sister J, great men think alike." The sister looked at him and said, "...and fools seldom differ."

21. "You are good-looking and smart."

I was working in Dumfries and Galloway. I lived in the doctor's accommodation which was within the hospital grounds. On one side of my accommodation was the main hospital and on the other side was the mental hospital. The hospital grounds had beautiful gardens and waterfalls and fountains.

One day after finishing my work I walked to the town centre for some shopping. As I was walking back, a woman in her 40s approached me, started talking to me and kept walking with me. She kept telling me how smart, good looking and attractive I was. I thought this woman was very lonely and probably wanted to talk to someone. I felt happy about what she was telling me. I thought when I go home; I would tease my wife that other women find me good looking, smart, and attractive.

The woman kept walking with me. As I entered the hospital grounds, she came in as well. I asked her why she was coming into the hospital, that too, in the evening.

She said that she was an inpatient in the mental hospital. She was not considered 'dangerous', so she was allowed to go anywhere. I asked her what she was doing in the town centre. She said that her eyesight was very weak, and she went to an optician.

When I told this whole incidence to my wife, she said: "Oh, yes, only the psychiatric patients with weak eyesight find you good-looking, smart and attractive." In reply, I told her: "No wonder why you fell in love with me, head over heels, when we first met."

22. "My baby is hungry…"

A woman was having a caesarean section under spinal analgesia, i.e., only the body below the ribs lose sensations, and otherwise, the patient is awake. We call the husband to sit next to the woman who is having the section.

This woman's husband came in and sat next to her. I was talking to the patient as well as to her husband. Everything went well and the baby was delivered without any complications. The baby was crying, which is quite normal. The woman was sent to the recovery room.

I came out of the theatres and went to the ward kitchen to make some coffee for myself. I saw the father of the baby in the kitchen, looking here and there. I asked him what he was looking for. He said, "My baby, just delivered, is crying; he must be hungry. I am looking for some toast for him."

23. Sleeping pills

A nurse was at the night ward rounds. By the time she reached the last patient, it was past midnight. The patient, an old man, was in a deep sleep and snoring. The nurse called the patient's name, but he did not wake up, as he was in a deep sleep. The nurse shook him, and then only he woke up and asked her what did she want? The nurse said, "Here are your sleeping pills."

24. What is wrong with your...

Three orthopaedic surgeons were standing outside a house. They saw a man limping and coming towards them. One surgeon said, "Oh, there is a problem with his hip bone." As the man came nearer, the second surgeon said, "No, there is something wrong with his knee." As the man came nearer, the third surgeon said to the other two surgeons, "Both of you are wrong...his ankle is sprained." When the man came near to them, they asked him what was wrong with him. The man replied, "My slippers are broken."

25. Psychiatrists

An airport wanted to improve the security at the airport. It employed a psychiatrist and told him to arrest anyone with suspicious behaviour. A few days later, they employed a second psychiatrist and gave him the same instructions. He arrested the first psychiatrist.

26. Is the cat married?

I was sitting in the doctor's sitting room with some of my colleagues. There was a newspaper nearby. I picked it up and started reading it. One of the news was that somebody had died and left two million pounds for his cat. I read this loudly. Then one of my friends asked me, "Oh, just see if that cat is married?" His wife was sitting next to him and she said, "Oh, I will be very happy if my husband marries that cat."

27. Psychology of desperation

This is just a joke and hopefully did not really happen.

A burglar broke into a house at night. The man and his wife woke up. The burglar took out his gun and said, "Since now, you two have seen me, you can identify me for the police. Therefore, I am going to kill you." Then he said, "I always ask the name of the person before I kill him/her, so what is your name?" He asked the wife. The wife said, "my name is Janet." The burglar kept quiet for a moment and said, "Sorry, I cannot kill you because my mum's name is Janet."

Then he asked the husband his name. The husband said, "Oh, well, when my mum was pregnant with me, she wished for a girl and when I was born, she refused to accept me as a boy, so she called me Janet. My name is Janet."

28. Looks are important

I was working in the Harrogate General Hospital (Harrogate, Yorkshire) as a junior doctor and was a resident in the hospital doctor's accommodation. It was a block of flats with many doctors living there.

One of the residents was an Egyptian lady doctor who was very particular about her looks. She was always very smartly dressed, full of makeup.

One night, as we were all sleeping in our rooms/flats, the fire alarm went off at around 2 am. Everyone woke up and started running outside, towards the open grounds, in their nightclothes.

The Egyptian lady doctor woke up. She was in her nightclothes. She changed into a very nice, smartly looking outfit, put the makeup on and then came out into the open grounds.

She saw everyone in their nightclothes, so she went back to her room, changed into her nice-looking nightgown, removed her makeup and then came down to the open grounds.

29. My trousers are falling

An orthopaedic surgeon was doing a hip replacement operation. Halfway through to the operation, he suddenly looked very uncomfortable. I asked him what the matter was. He said, "Oh, my trousers are falling." He was scrubbed, so he could not stop his trousers from falling. Someone else had to do it. All the nurses in the operation theatre were female and they refused to hold and tie his trousers. Without my liking, I was 'honoured' to do the job.

30. Wrong changing room?

I was working in a hospital in the north of England. On my first day, after finishing the operation theatre session, I went to the changing room to change into my normal clothes.

A female nurse walked in and started changing in front of me. I told her that that was a male changing room. She smiled and asked me if I was new to the hospital. I said yes. Then she said: "In these theatres, there is only one changing room. Men and women change in the same room." After this, I had no choice but to get used to it.

31. OK, no problem

In the Medway hospital, Gillingham, Kent, I was doing an orthopaedic case in the A & E (Accident and Emergencies). I had a male junior trainee doctor with me. Towards the end of the procedure, while the patient was still unconscious, a young female plaster technician came in to put the plaster on the patient's arm. She was wearing a low-neck blouse. As she was bending down to put the plaster, her low-neck blouse became more low neck, and my young junior male trainee doctor, instead of concentrating on his work, kept looking down her blouse. I told her that her low-neck blouse was distracting my assistant. She said, "OK, no problem", took her blouse off, then and there, turned it around and wore it.

I could see the disappointment on my junior's face.

32. Oh no, please don't drink.

I was in the coffee room of the operation theatres with other colleagues, waiting for the patient. A lady gynaecologist Miss J was there as well.

A porter walked in and started making a cup of tea for himself. Then he asked Miss J if she wanted a cup of tea. She said, "Yes." The porter took another mug, took the tea bag, made the cup of tea, put the sugar, and gave it to Miss J. She was about to drink the tea when I jolted her arm purposely and the tea fell on the floor. She looked at me with a questioning face. I ignored her. Other people present in the coffee room were surprised as well. The porter had just left. Then I told Miss J that this porter, like quite a few other people, including some doctors, when they go to the toilet, after they finish the 'job', big or small, they walk off without washing their hands. I was in the changing room when this porter used the toilet and then came to the coffee room, without washing his hands and made tea for himself and for Miss J. This was the reason I jolted her hand and made the tea drop on the floor. Miss J. was very grateful to me.

I told the theatre manager about people not washing their hands after using the toilet. He said he could not do anything about this issue except to put a big notice in the toilet: 'Please wash your hands'. This notice was already there in every toilet.

33. Five camels

In the 1980s, I was working at Bethnal Green Hospital in East London.

In the operation theatres, there was an English nurse, quite pretty and quite friendly. An Arab doctor arrived to work in the hospital and became quite friendly with me. The first time he had left home and therefore was feeling very homesick.

One afternoon, as I was having lunch in the hospital canteen, the Arab doctor was with me as well. The English nurse came and joined me (us) for lunch. I introduced the Arab doctor to this nurse.

The next day, the nurse in the theatre looked at me and started laughing. I asked her why she was laughing. She said that my Arab friend fell in love with her at first sight and offered her 'five camels' if she would marry her.

The next day, I told her (bluffed in a joke) that I had talked to the carpark manager of the hospital and he was happy to make room, in the carpark, for five camels.

34. See you later

This is a common phrase in English when two people are parting from each other.

In the Medway hospital, Kent, England, a Burmese lady doctor, Dr B, was recruited at a junior post in the operating department. She was very new to the UK. Her English was not that great.

On the first day of her job, my consultant told me to take her around the hospital, show her the various departments and various protocols/procedures etc. She was struggling with her English language. The whole procedure of 'showing her around' took some time. In the end, when we were parting, I said to her, "Thank you very much, I will see you later."

I went back to my room in the hospital. A few hours later, I went to the switchboard to change the batteries in my bleep. The lady operator told me, "What have you done to Dr B? She came here to talk to me. She has been crying since you left her. She does not want to go back to her room. She is scared of you." When I enquired in detail, she thought I was going to see her later that night, to spend the night with her. This is what she understood by the phrase 'See you later'.

35. Someone…somebody

Working as a junior doctor in the early 1980s in Medway hospital, Gillingham, Kent, England, one day I went to the operation theatre at 8 a.m., finished around 6:30 p.m., rested a bit in the theatres and then went to the surgical ward to see the patients, we had operated on that day.

The nurse's station was empty. Nurses were either on their break or busy in the ward. I was alone at the station, looking at the notes of the patient.

I saw a man looking here and there eagerly and anxiously. I asked him and he said he was looking for someone. Then he told me to let him know if I found someone. Then he disappeared. I did not ask his name or the name of the person he was looking for. So, I left a note for the nurses, just to tease them, which said:

"Somebody is looking for someone; when you find someone, please tell somebody."

36. Neighbours

In a UK hospital, a young boy, about 17 years old, was admitted, having a surgical procedure.

I went to the ward to see him before his surgery. He asked me what time his operation was. I said 2 p.m.

He made a big fuss about it. He wanted his operation either first thing in the morning or very late in the afternoon. I asked him why? His reply was:

"I don't want to miss *Neighbours* (the famous Australian soap on TV)."

We had to readjust the order of the operating list, which caused quite a bit of inconvenience for all of us (instruments issues, availability of beds, etc.). He was a day-care patient, due to go home that evening, but because his operation was done last on the list, we could not send him home; we had to find a bed for him for an overnight stay.

Q: Is the NHS taken for granted?

37. Fantastic, beautiful

Doing any kind of work, day in day out, one gets used to it and talks about it casually, no matter how disgusting it is.

In a doctors' sitting room in a hospital in England, I heard this conversation between two doctors call them A (Registrar in gastroenterology) and B (Registrar in respiratory medicine). They both were doing some research/audit work in their specialities:

B to A: "How is your audit going on? Did you manage to get some decent samples of vomit and faeces?"

A: "Yes and No. Only one patient vomited nicely. I was there, so I managed to get all his vomit in the bowl. Oh, such a decent and fantastic vomit, beautiful. The other two patients did not do so well. Their vomits were not as good as I expected, so I am waiting for some more patients to vomit, hopefully, I will get some nice, smelly, bile-coated vomit."

B: "How about faecal samples? Any luck there?"

A: "Oh yes, I got what I wanted, five very nice, blood-coated samples of faeces. I can't ask for any more... lovely and beautiful.

How about you? How is your audit and research going on about the sputum of patients with chronic bronchitis? Did you manage to get some nice green sputum?"

B: "Oh yes, I got all the samples I wanted. They are nice and smelly."

38. I don't have the right equipment

I was doing a C-section with my consultant (a Scottish gentleman), in a London hospital.

When the baby came out, he was crying quite loudly. He was in the standard incubator, still crying. My consultant took him in his arms and started walking up and down in the theatre, trying to calm down the baby. The baby kept crying.

The nurse, standing by, told my consultant that the baby was hungry and needed to be fed.

The consultant, smiling, looked down at his chest, under his theatre blues, and giving the baby to the nurse he said, "I don't have the right equipment to feed the baby; you feed him... You seem to have the big equipment."

Everyone laughed; the nurse took it lightly.

39. Assisted conception

In a London hospital, a fair amount of work was being done for the artificial methods of conception like IVF, etc. I was an active member of the team. The department was signposted as 'Assisted conception'.

One day I was coming out of the resuscitation room and I had a medical student with me.

Passing by the 'Assisted conception' signpost, the student asked me, "What is assisted conception?"

I was in a light-hearted mood, so I gave him an explanation which I should not write here. I thought he would pick up that I was joking. To my surprise, he believed in everything I said.

When we reached the operation theatre coffee room, I made a cup of coffee for him and gave him the real explanation of what is assisted conception and told him that I was just joking.

Working in the acute specialities of the hospital work, doctors, from time to time, need to release the tension and go into a light-hearted mood.

40. Dining table/dissection table (1961)

In my medical school in Hyderabad, India, I, like other medical students, spent two years in the anatomy dissection hall.

The attendees there used to look after dead bodies. They had a busy job and did not always get time to go out for lunch. At times like these, they would open their tiffin box, put it on the dissection table, use it as a dining table and have their lunch. A few inches from their food, a dead body was lying, half dissected with its chest, abdomen opened and arms and legs dissected.

I am sure things have changed by now. At that time, it did look funny.

Chapter Twenty-Two
Miscellaneous Topics (Mainly on Psychology) of General Interest

Introduction

In the 1950s and 60s and even before this time, in the Indian subcontinent, mental illness was a stigma. People accepted and showed sympathy if someone's liver, heart or stomach etc., were diseased. However, diseases of mind (mental illness) were not looked at with the same sympathy. Anxiety, depression, mood swings, aggression, frustration, suicidal tendencies etc., were not regarded as mental illness but, they all had other explanations, i.e., straight away, the diagnosis was that the person was possessed by evil forces. The reasons for these possessions were very strange, for example: the person urinated under a tree which was the dwelling place of a Jinn (spirit), which upsets the Jinn or, the girl came out in the evening, with open hair (sign of attractiveness) and a Jinn fell in love with her, etc. Women were more affected by mental illness probably because of the effects of monthly periods, pregnancy, delivery, postnatal depression, menopause, domestic abuse, poverty, husbands' interest outside marriages, etc.

but the diagnosis was, 'possessed by Jinn'.

Because of these reasons, psychiatry was not a money-making speciality for doctors in their private practice. Nobody would go to psychiatrists; they would rather go to a "saint" who would "kick out" the Jinn with his exorcism. It was a good money-making trick for the saints. I have seen such exorcism acts in India and Pakistan.

In my six years of medical education and training in India, I had six months to one-year postings in specialities like General Medicine, General Surgery, orthopaedics, E.N.T., Eye, Obstetrics and Gynaecology etc., but only ten days of exposure in a mental hospital.

When I came to the UK, one of the things I was involved, was the ECT (Electro-Convulsive Therapy) in the psychiatric wards. In this procedure, controlled electric shock is given to the patient's head in a controlled environment. The whole body goes into convulsions. The more severe the convulsions are, the better are the results of the treatment. For each patient, this treatment goes on for weeks to months. The indications for ECT are variable and include chronic depression not responding to medical treatment, Bipolar disorders etc.

In the early days of ECT treatment, there had been cases where the convulsions used to be so severe that in some patients, it broke the jaw and backbones (vertebrae). These days it is very safe, thanks to the advances in Anaesthetics. No patient I was involved with ended up with broken bones due to ECT.

Although psychology/psychiatry is not my speciality, reading the notes of the patients coming for the ECT treatment, I got interested in psychology and psychiatry.

I did my own studies as to why does the human mind get diseased. As we can take preventive measures for physical illness, for example, with dieting and exercise, we can prevent/reduce diseases of heart, diabetes, high blood pressure, cancer etc., and with vaccinations, we can prevent bacterial and viral diseases including Covid-19, with anti-malarial tablets, we can prevent malaria etc., can we take any preventive measures for mental illness? To find the answer to my question :

I read various books on psychology, American and Asian, watched some programmes on TV and combined them with the knowledge of religions. My view is that a sensible approach to religion plays an important role in creating a stable mind. Right religious teachings (not extremism), upbringing, childhood, socio-economic status, surroundings at home and outside, and level of education are the preventative measures for the development of mental illness.

Saying that religion plays an important role in the creation of a stable mind, I know quite a few people in the local mosque who do have mental illness. They consult me about the side effects of the drugs they are taking. These people are the regular attendees of the mosque. They are regarded as "religious" people. So, is my theory wrong? i.e., religion plays an important role in preventing mental illnesses.

The answer is No. Being religious, doing the rituals, adopting a certain appearance, etc., is quite different from understanding the teachings of religion. The general principles of all the religions are same. So, regardless of what is your religion, if you understand its message, you should not have any mental illness.

Example: **1.** I know a Muslim lady here in London whose husband died. She got so shocked and distressed that she stopped believing in God. She was angry with God, and she kept saying: "How can this happen to me? I refuse to believe that he is dead", etc.

Example: **2.** In India, my best friend in the medical school was an orthodox Hindu, a Brahmin. I was the only Muslim allowed in his house. When his brother-in-law (sister's husband) died in an accident, his father stopped worshipping all gods. He showed the same reaction as that of the Muslim lady. He could not bear the sight of his young daughter, who was going to spend the rest of her life as a widow.

Example: 3. Here in London, in a Muslim family, person A was a chain smoker all his life. He died of lung cancer. His brother B was shocked by the death and went into a depression to such an extent that he started ignoring his wife and children. This went on for some time. Mrs B got so upset with the behaviour of her husband that when I visited them to offer my condolence, she asked me: "Why did Allah not ban cigarettes and tobacco in the Quran?"

Here again, the problem is not understanding the religion.

Although tobacco and cigarettes are not mentioned in the Quran, there is a verse that says: "Do *not do anything with your own hands that will destroy you.*" Surah 2, verse 195. If A had known this verse and followed its practice, he would have kept away from cigarettes.

Example 4: I had a personal encounter with the three examples given above, but this 4th one, I read in a book of true incidences.

Person "A" had a daughter, his only child. In her teenage, she met a violent death due to the wrong company. "A" was so shocked; he kept shouting, "who is great? Allah or death" He kept repeating it and went into an incredibly angry mood, taking out his anger on everyone. It was not known if he came back to "normal" after the initial shock or not. The reason for not knowing this was that he died two months after his daughter's death.

With correct religious teaching, the reaction to acute mental trauma will be less severe.

Every religion teaches to be patient, tolerant and have self-control under stressful conditions. The Arabic word for these qualities is "Sabar".

In a Hadith, The Prophet said: "The real Sabar(patience) is at the time of the acute phase of a trauma/ unpleasant event." In the Quran, this word has come many times and the reward for having Sabar at the time of calamity is enormous.

Going back to the examples above, the people involved showed the typical psychological reaction of severe emotional trauma. The reaction is:

D A D A.
Denial, Anger, Depression, Acceptance.

In severe emotional trauma, generally the victim first denies that it happened to him, then he gets angry with God and with people around him, then he goes into depression. Finally, the reality sets in and he accepts it.

All religions teach that death is a fact of life but not the end of life. Problems are part of life but not the end of life. One, who understands this, will accept death/problems as one of the laws of nature (God), which is non-negotiable, like all the other laws of nature. It is natural to feel sad, but life must go on. Such people, when they do not come out of depression, despite medical treatment, are the candidates for E.C.T.

Throughout this book and in this chapter as well, as a Muslim, I have quoted verses from Holy Quran and other books on Islam, but people of other beliefs can also find the same kind of teaching in their scriptures, as the general principles of all the religions are same.

Some selected topics

1: Negative Feelings

Feelings can be physical or mental.

The mental feelings are to experience or sense an emotion, like, "I feel very down", "I feel happy", "She was over the moon", he was angry, etc. These feelings can be positive or negative or sometimes neutral.

Positive feelings are good for the mind and body. The negative feelings are not. In our everyday life, we all have positive and negative feelings. Having negative feelings all the time, over a period, can cause "psychosomatic disorders". Examples are stress-related illnesses like stomach ulcers, diabetes, heart conditions etc.

Jealousy, animosity, anger, frustration, ill feelings, anxiety, fear, fear of the unknown, depression and sometimes hatred towards others, not being content with life, being ungrateful to God, comparison and competition with others are natural negative feelings. In this and as in everything in life, there is a test for us. To my understanding, this is the teaching of all religions. In fact, the purpose of life is "TEST", as is mentioned in this verse of the Quran.

"He (Allah) created life and death to test which of you are best in deeds." **(Al-Mulk, Surah 67, verse 2).**

When you get these negative feelings towards your creator or towards any person, think of all the good things God has given to you; think of other things in which you are blessed. Almost certainly, you will find many. Then be grateful to God. Thinking of all the good things you have in life creates positive feelings. Quran has many verses which encourage positive thinking. Like

"Rehearse and proclaim all the good things We have given to you" **(Surah 93, verse 11).** The other one is, "Whatever problems you have in life, face them with boldness, courage and consistency. Indeed, doing so is a great thing." **(Surah 31, verse 17)**

If you are not happy with what you have in life and comparing yourself with others, then remember this verse:

"Do not desire something in which Allah has preferred others over you." **(Surah 4, verse 32).** What this means is that Allah may prefer someone over you in somethings, but He may prefer you over the other person in something else. You should remember all the things in which Allah has preferred you over others rather than focus on what you don't have. Allah does this is to keep a balance in the worldly affairs.

If you consider carefully, almost certainly, you will find that you have something which others do not have. To start with, you should not be in a "comparative "mode. However, it is natural to "feel" if someone has more than you. While comparing with others, do not just be confined with material things. You may have happiness at home, which others, very rich people, with whom you are comparing yourself, may not have. Even if this does not help you, then think of this verse: *"Whatever you have in this world will perish, and what you leave (good deeds) with Allah will remain." (Surah 16, verse 96).*

There are Prophetic sayings (Ahadith) on this topic as well, e.g., "Best of the contentment is the content of the heart".

Similarly, if you have such negative feelings towards other human beings because he/she has done something wrong to you, think of at least one good thing that person has done for you. This approach is particularly helpful when an argument/quarrel starts between husband and wife. There are Ahadith on this topic as well, which basically say that "see the good points in your spouse rather than thinking of all the wrong/ bad things he/she has or has done."

If a person has achieved something with his own hard work and you did not (because you have not worked for it), remember, God is fair and just. He has some set, fundamental rules to run this world. One of these rules is:

"If you work for it, you will get it", (Surah 53, verse 39).

2: Social relationships.

A human being cannot live alone. He needs other human beings for his physical, social, mental, and other needs. A relationship develops between him and others. However, this relationship is not always perfect. To make it as perfect as possible, the following points may be helpful:

R A T T L H E FFL, D and D before C.

Here are the details of these letters:

1. **Respect**: Every human being expects and deserves respect. If you do not give due respect to the person, either he will move away from you if he does not need you, or if he is under you, depends on you, and cannot move away from you (your employee, wife, and children), then he will hate you from inside. Once he is independent and powerful, he will move away from you or even take revenge for how you had treated him in the past. The worst you can do is to insult him in the presence of others. This wound never heals. I know few people in India who insulted and humiliated their wives, throughout their lives, in the presence of their

children. Poor wives could not do much. When children grew up, they hated their fathers. When those people died, the wives celebrated their deaths.

I also knew some people who, in their childhood, received not just the beatings but also the most insulting and humiliating treatments from their fathers, that too, in the presence of others. Now, grown-up, they have not forgotten how their fathers had treated them. After the deaths of their fathers, when they were told to pray for the fathers, their answer was, "It should come from my heart. I cannot force myself to pray for my father".

They also said that the pain of beatings had gone, but the feelings of helplessness, being lowest of the low and the fear, the inferiority complex is created in them, the insult and humiliation they felt, had not gone and affected their personalities, and their progress in life. Physical wounds heal, living scars, visible to everyone. Mental wounds do not heal, even if the scars they leave are not visible to everyone, but their effects are reflected in their personalities.

Good manners are the parts of respect.

2. **Appreciation:** It is a human desire to be appreciated for the good things he has or he does. This creates a positive feeling in him. It gives "worth" to his existence. This rule of appreciation should be applied everywhere, at home, at work and anywhere else.

At home, when the wife/ husband does anything nice each deserves appreciation. It is a satisfaction to her/him to be appreciated.

When children do anything well, appreciate them, encourage them. It boosts their confidence and creates love for you. They feel that you take an interest in their affairs.

At work, when your junior colleagues or your employees do good things, again appreciate them. In return, they develop respect, love, and loyalty for you. These are the commodities you cannot buy with money.

3. **Trust:** A very important ingredient in social life, especially so between husband and wife. Trust takes some time to build up but can be blown up in a very short time.

Trust your children as well. Trust in their abilities, in their truthfulness etc. They appreciate this and it builds up their confidence.

At work, trust your colleagues, especially the juniors who work with you. It is good for them and good for you.

Use common sense when trusting others. Blind belief or blind trust can be harmful.

4. Tolerance: We all have shortfalls. Nobody is perfect. To err is human. When this happens at home, with wife, or children, or at work with colleagues, show patience and tolerance. You cannot "hit the roof" for every little thing that has gone wrong, but if you do, they can also do the same when you do something "not nice". If they are not "allowed" to do so (usually wives and children), they will hate you from the inside of their hearts.

5. Love: To love and to be loved is a human desire. Your wife and children expect love from you. Just loving them in your heart is not enough. You need to express this. This expression does not have to be in the form of expensive presents. A smile, few words of appreciation, a tap on the shoulder or a hug can mean a lot.

Outside the family, love can be expressed with good manners, some gifts and helping them in need.

6. Help: When you can, you should help others. A friend in need is a friend indeed. This has a long-lasting effect on the minds of those whom you helped in their need. This gives you satisfaction as well. However, it is important not to "emotionally" torture the person you helped by reminding him of what you did for him. Nor you go round telling others of the favour you did for the person.

At the same time, you should not be exploited either. Make a sensible judgment, to help or not and how much to help.

7. Expectations: Do not have "too much", "unrealistic", or "unreasonable" expectations from others, especially from your life partner. Otherwise, you will be hurt and your behaviour towards that person will change. Be

realistic; you cannot fulfil all the expectations others have from you, so why have expectations from them?

8. **Forgive and Forget.** It is the best principle to heal past and present wounds. All the religions of the world teach "forgiveness".

9. **Limits.** Every person is an individual. He/she lives in an invisible case around him/her. This is "his/her" space. Do not enter into this space. In other words:

Know your limits. Depending on your relations with the person, these limits can be variable. For example, between my wife and me, we can open each other's letters, e-mails, texts etc. This is not the case with every couple. For them, it is a matter of "interference with the privacy. No matter how close you are to a person, there are still some limits you need to observe. It is like "keep your distance" signs on Motorways (highways). If you do not keep the distance, the chances of an accident are high. Similarly, if you do not observe your limits with another person, albeit your wife, the chances of a conflict are high.

After putting every advice written above into practice, if any dispute arises between you and others, then the best policy is:

10. **D and D** before **C**: This stands for **D**ialogue and **D**iplomacy before Confrontation. In family life, with friends and at work, disputes do arise. Most of these can be sorted out by **D and D.**

In my working life and at home, I have used this principle quite successfully, many times.

If you end up in a confrontation, try to do the minimum or no damage to the other person. There should be no collateral damage because of your confrontation. For example, your employee is not doing very well. Sacking him should be the last resort because sacking will cause collateral damage to his family.

The Prophet (PBUH) has put some rules of the war. In all the disputes, he tried D and D before C. For C, his rules were: No attack on the enemy when his back is towards you, when he is unarmed, when he is accompanied by women and children, and when he is fleeing from the battlefield. No collateral damage in the form of burning the houses and farms, slaughtering livestock, kidnapping the children, or assaulting women in any form.

In everyday life, this principle will keep you happy.

You will win the peace before winning the war.

3. Treatment with children.

Warm and Permissive against Cold and Restrictive

Bringing up children and training them to be good humans is a task. The above four letters say what to do and what not to do.

Your behaviour with children should be **Warm and P**ermissive and not **C**old and **R**estrictive.

Children brought up in a warm and permissive atmosphere do much better in life than those brought up in a cold and restrictive atmosphere. They are creative, bold, intelligent, and sensible with all positive thoughts.

Children in the other category (cold and restrictive) do not achieve much in life and go towards a life of crimes.

"Warm" behaviour means showing love, affection, respect, encouragement and all such positive points. Cool behaviour is opposite to this.

Permissiveness is a relative term, and it should be adjusted to your personal believes and culture. For example, as a Muslim, I was permissive to my children, i.e., let them do what they wanted to do, but not to the extent that I allowed them to drink alcohol and do other things forbidden in Islam.

4. Stable home: Man and wife, following the above rules should be able to establish a healthy, stable home and with this a happy married life and bright future for children.

If you are not happy at home, you cannot do something great in the outer world.

As a child in India, I knew many children who, at the end of their school, did not want to go home. Their fathers were responsible for creating hell at home.

There are men, who at the end of their working day, do not want to go home (husband and wife not getting on well).

Note: What I have written above is extracted from various books on psychology and Behavioural sciences combined with religious knowledge.

5. Problems are part of life.

Life without problems is fine, but it deprives you of the knowledge and experience you gain when you have problems and deal with them.

When God made this world and humans, He set certain rules to run the world and its affairs. We can call these "Laws of nature". Nobody is an exemption to these rules. For example, we all feel hungry and thirsty, fall ill, have social and other problems. No one is exempted, neither the Prophets of Allah, nor the kings, nor the beggars. Similarly, problems are part of the laws of nature.

What to do?

Follow the general principles of whatever your religion is. They are all the same. They are:

Patience, tolerance, perseverance, steadfastness, be grateful to what you have, etc. Follow the examples of the pious people given in your religious books.

Running away from a problem is not the solution to the problem. Take up the challenge and face it boldly, especially so if you are the leader of a nation or a group of people, or a boss at work or bringing up your family. or. In times of stress, everyone looks at you and expects you to sort out the problem.

****

There are many more topics and a lot more to write about. It may be in part 2.

The End